ESSENTIAL
ANATOMY

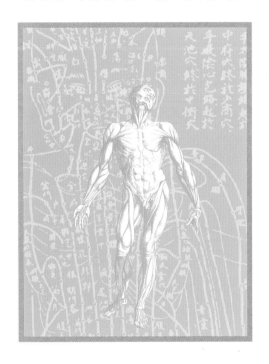

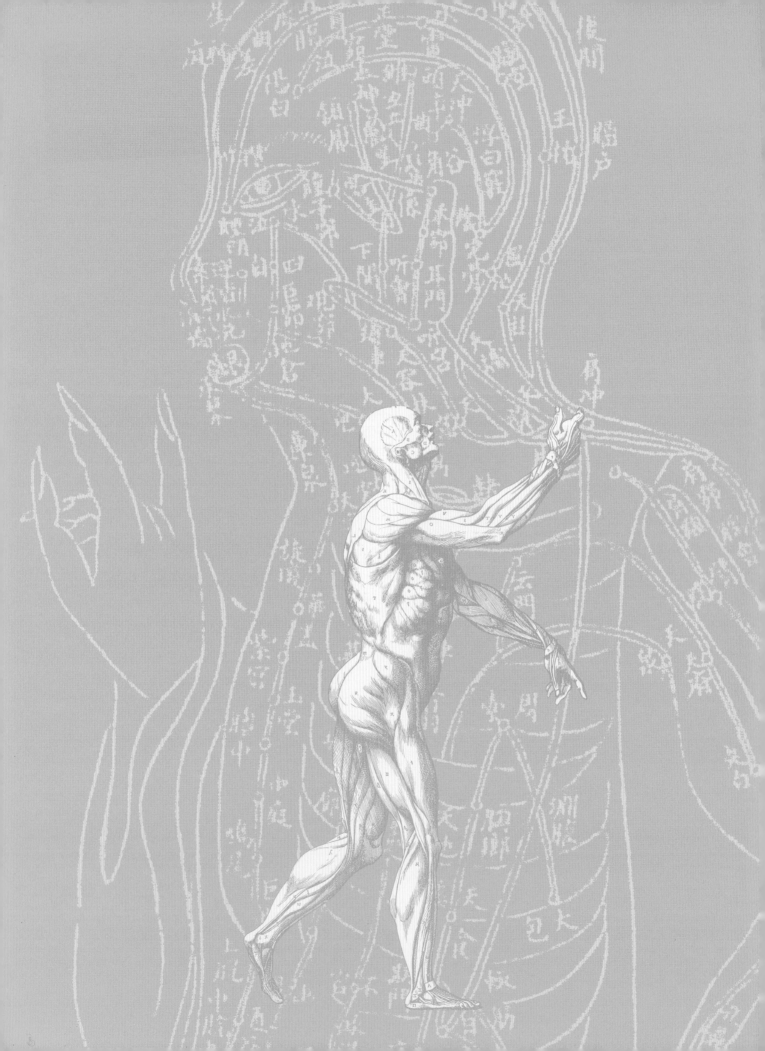

ESSENTIAL ANATOMY

For Healing & Martial Arts

M A R C   T E D E S C H I

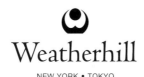

Weatherhill

NEW YORK • TOKYO

FIRST EDITION, 2000

08 07 06 05 04 03 02 01 00   5 4 3 2 1

Book and cover design: Marc Tedeschi
Photography: Frank Deras, Shelley Firth
Creative consultant: Michele Wetherbee
Editorial supervision: Thomas Tedeschi
Chinese typesetting: Birdtrack Press
Printing and binding: Leefung-Asco
Set in Helvetica Neue, Univers, Sabon, and Weiss.

Library of Congress Cataloging-in-Publication Data
Tedeschi, Marc.
   Essential anatomy for healing and martial arts /
   Marc Tedeschi.—1st ed.
      p. cm.
   Includes index.
   ISBN 0-8348-0443-3 (alk. paper)
   1. Acupuncture points. 2. Human anatomy.
   3. Martial arts. 4. Healing. I. Title
RM184.5.T43 2000
615.8'92—dc21   99-086253

Notice of Liability
The information in this book is distributed without warranty. All information and techniques are to be used at the reader's sole discretion. While every precaution has been taken in preparation of this book, neither the author nor publisher shall have any liability to any person or entity with respect to liability, loss, or damage caused or alleged to be caused directly or indirectly by the contents contained in this book or by the procedures or processes described herein. There is no guarantee that the techniques described or shown in this book will be safe or effective in any medical or self-defense situation, or otherwise. The information in this book is not intended as a substitute for qualified medical advice. You may be injured if you apply or train in the martial techniques described in this book. Consult a physician regarding whether or not to attempt any technique described in this book. Specific self-defense responses illustrated in this book may not be justified in any particular situation in view of all of the circumstances or under the applicable federal, state or local laws.

Acknowledgments

The quality of this book was immeasurably strengthened by the love, support and creative contributions of my close friends, in particular Shelley Firth, Michele Wetherbee and Frank Deras. I am also indebted to my editor at Weatherhill, Ray Furse, who had the vision and energy to make this project a reality. I would also like to thank Thomas Tedeschi for editing the majority of the book; Jeffrey Hunter for clarifying Japanese translations; and Charlie Goldberg, M.D., Tieh Chun Wang, M.D., and Jo-An Aguirre, R.N. for reviewing the manuscript and sharing their insightful comments. The following individuals graciously donated their time to appear in the photographs: Jo-An Aguirre (revival techniques), Kathryn Kidney (massage techniques), and Arnold Dungo and Cody Aguirre (martial techniques). Finally, I would like to express my gratitude to all those individuals and teachers too numerous to mention, who unselfishly shared their wisdom and experiences with me—without which I would never have found my way in this life.

CONTENTS

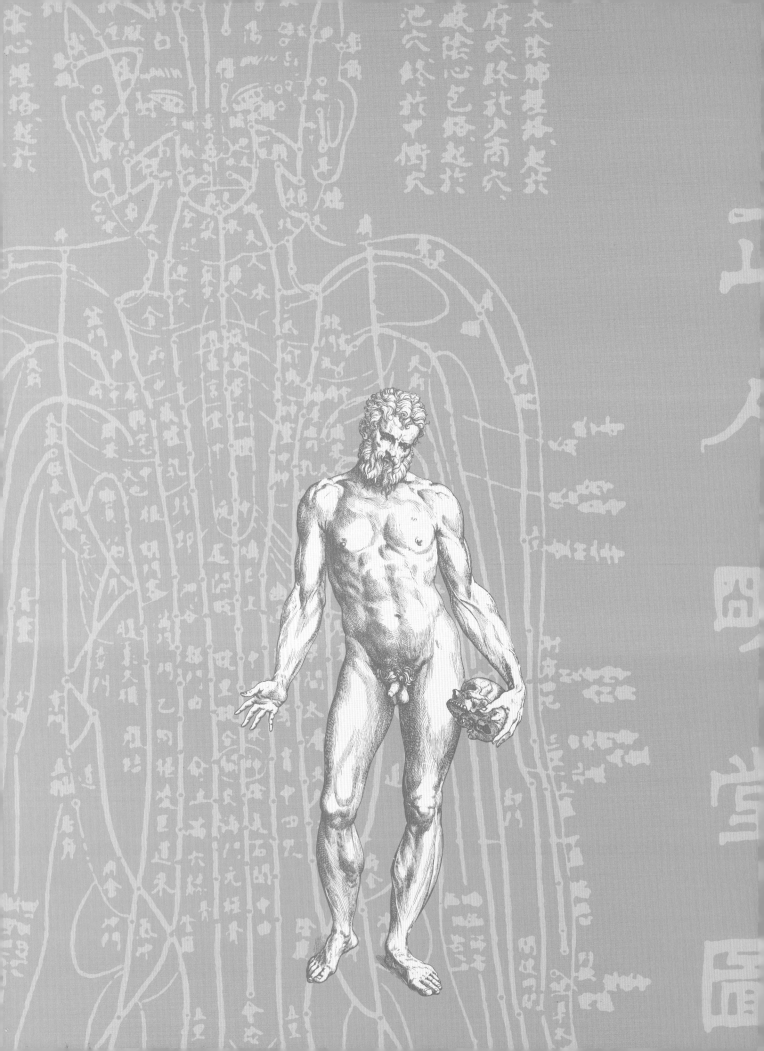

The purpose of this book is to familiarize martial artists and healing practitioners with basic concepts of the human body, as defined by both Western and Eastern healing traditions. In contemporary approaches to the martial and healing arts, a fundamental understanding of both of these medical traditions is extremely valuable, since they provide differing yet complementary points of view. Western medicine, with its emphasis on the modern scientific method, has allowed us to understand in a very

OVERVIEW

material way how our bodies work, or don't work. In contrast, traditional Eastern medicine, with its emphasis on a 3000 year old philosophical tradition, has helped us to comprehend a more holistic and energetic concept of the human body—one which Western science is only beginning to grasp. By studying these traditions collectively, perhaps we can come to a more complete, holistic, and scientifically forward-looking view of the body—one which truly enriches our practice of the martial and healing arts.

For martial artists and healing practitioners, knowledge of human anatomy is vitally important, since it greatly influences the effectiveness of both martial and healing techniques. Limited knowledge results in crude, ineffectual techniques that expend much energy; while extensive knowledge yields highly efficient and effective skills. For example, detailed knowledge of pressure points can be used to magnify the effect of strikes or holds, or accelerate the healing of injuries. This book will outline essential anatomical principles, body functions and vital targets, in both Eastern and Western medical systems—both of which have value to martial artists and healers.

Concepts of the Human Body

There are various systems for classifying and understanding the human body. Western medicine tends to be based upon the study of body structures, scientific observation, and the analysis of quantifiable phenomena. This has led to a systemic concept in which the body is made up of various major systems, such as the nervous system, circulatory system, skeletal system, etc.

Traditional Eastern medicine is deeply rooted in ancient philosophical systems and views the body in an entirely different manner. For example, there is no concept of a nervous system, and only a general concern for anatomical structure. Rather, the human body is seen as a complex of life-sustaining processes, preserved and nourished by the circulation of *essential fluids* and *vital energy*. While individual Eastern cultures have evolved their own unique medical traditions, they all nonetheless embody this fundamental idea.

For example, the medical traditions of China, Korea and Japan view the human body as a complex network of *meridians,* which are paths for distributing *vital energy* (called *Qi*) to specific areas of the body. At various places the meridians run close to the surface of the body. Located along these paths are small external points, commonly called *acupoints*, which can be used to regulate the flow of Qi.

In Eastern medicine, acupoints are manipulated by massage, acupuncture or other healing procedures, in an effort to maintain or restore health. In martial arts, these same points are attacked to increase the effectiveness of strikes, blocks, holds and throws.

The medical and philosophical traditions of India also purport a similar energetic concept of the human body. This is reflected in disciplines such as Ayurvedic medicine and yoga, in which the human body is thought to comprise seven major energy centers, called *Chakras*, which are supported by a complex of minor Chakras. The Chakras interact to regulate vital energy (called *Prana*), controlling and defining all of the body's life-sustaining processes. Prana circulates throughout the body along paths called *Nadis*. In traditional Indian medicine, all the qualities and actions in one's life are seen as factors affecting health and vitality.

Some Comparisons

The difference between Eastern and Western systems can be better understood by looking at a few examples: Eastern medicine recognizes a relationship between specific acupoints on the body's surface, and specific internal physiological functions. For instance, inserting acupuncture needles into specific acupoints on the arm can lower blood pressure. Western medicine finds no physical justification for this, although theories outlining the material basis of Eastern medicine have been postulated for decades.

Energetic Terms: *Throughout history, many terms have evolved to describe the fundamental life-force or energy that animates all living things. Some are:*

Astral Light	Huna	Paraelectricity
Arealoha	Ka	Pneuma
Archeus	Kerei	Prana
Baraka	Mana	Reiki
Bioenergy	Mumia	Spiritus
Bioplasma	Mungo	Syntropy
Chi, Qi, Ki	Nervous Ether	Tinh
Eckankar	Numen	Tondi
Elima	Odic Force	Vis Naturalis
God	Orenda	Wakan

Currently, high blood pressure is usually treated with drugs which effect changes in the circulatory and nervous systems.

Another, martial, example: In Western terms, a *knockout* may be caused by a forceful strike to the head, violently slamming the brain against the skull cavity wall. This is called a concussion and is the result of trauma to the brain. Eastern martial techniques can also produce unconsciousness by lightly striking a series of key acupoints on the trunk or extremities. There is no proven *scientific* explanation of this effect, although acupoint strikes have produced consistent observable results for centuries. Both striking techniques work. The second method requires much less power, but a great deal more accuracy, skill and knowledge.

While Eastern and Western systems may appear quite different, they nonetheless view many of the same areas and points as vital or extremely sensitive. For example, sensitive points along the ulnar and median nerves correspond to acupoints on the Heart and Pericardium meridians. In the martial and healing arts, how such points are identified is not nearly as important as knowing where they are, what they affect, and how they are manipulated to produce specific results.

Whether certain techniques work as a result of modifications to neural impulses, changes in electromagnetic fields, biochemical changes, or manipulation of acupoints affecting Qi-flow or bioenergy is, for our purposes, largely irrelevant. Martial artists are more concerned with the result than with the specific medical or philosophical reasons behind it. When they strike someone, it is with a specific purpose in mind (deter, immobilize, kill). The better they can predict and control the outcome of a technique, the better off they are, and the more control they have in a given situation. Many healers share a similar viewpoint: they are more interested in engendering successful, life-affirming treatments, than understanding the precise scientific mechanisms at work.

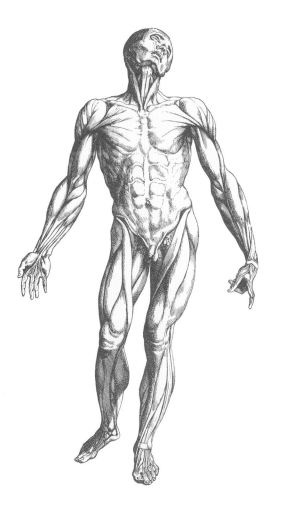

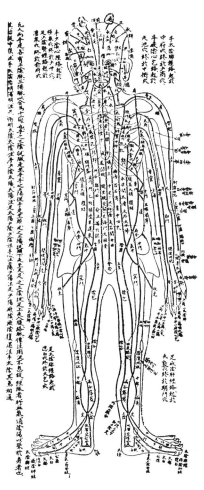

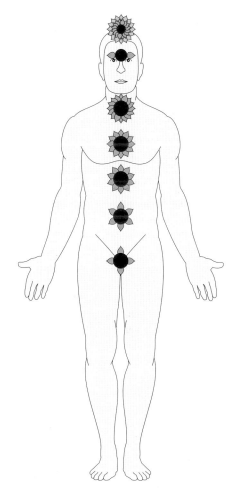

Left: Western scientific concept of the human body as made up of interrelated systems of muscles, tissues, bones, nerves, blood vessels, cells, and organs.

The drawing shown was done by Vesalius in the 16th century, and is based on anatomical observations obtained by dissection of the human body.

Center: Eastern philosophical concept of the human body as a complex network of meridians, which are pathways for distributing vital energy, called Qi.

The drawing shown is a meridian map dating from 200 BC. Ancient Eastern healers did not concern themselves with the actual physical makeup of the body.

Right: Indian spiritual concept of the human body as a complex of energy centers and channels that distribute vital energy, called Prana, throughout the body.

The drawing shown is a modern depiction. While India possesses many ancient medical texts, it has virtually no ancient tradition of illustrative medical drawings.

The Evolution of Healing Arts

Most historians agree that the world's great healing traditions emerged gradually during the same period of time, predominantly in China, India and the Mediterranean. All of these great traditions evolved as an intimate reflection of the spiritual and philosophical practices of their native cultures. While this has led to many unique approaches to medicine, it should be realized that none of these healing traditions developed in isolation. They all influenced one another to various degrees, usually as part of the larger cultural interactions of the times—religious, philosophical, scientific and combative.

Indian medical traditions migrated with Buddhism into Southeast and Central Asia. Chinese medical knowledge spread into neighboring regions such as Korea, Japan, and the Indochinese peninsula. Native Tibetan medicine emerged during the seventh century, by blending Indian medical concepts with Chinese and other foreign influences; it was then transmitted to Mongolia a millennium later. The Western Greco-Roman medical tradition, which was embraced by the Arab-Islamic world after the seventh century, found its way into India via the Islamic conquests. In fact, Western medicine shared many of the naturalistic and element-oriented concepts commonly associated with Eastern medicine until the seventeenth century, when it rapidly departed down the road of rationalism and science. So as one can see, all of these unique healing traditions have influenced one another to some degree. As a result, one often notes points of similarity.

The Future: One World View?

In past decades, it has been common for many writers to portray Eastern and Western medicine as two completely different entities, with diametrically opposed viewpoints. While there is a certain element of historical truth in this, one must also understand that there is a clear difference between "traditional" and "contemporary" Eastern medicine. While both approaches are actively employed throughout East Asia, one might be surprised to learn that the average Chinese hospital utilizes more Western medical procedures than traditional Eastern procedures. This is not surprising, since many Eastern medical traditions evolved by assimilating influences from a variety of outside cultures. As contact with the West increased, traditional Taoist and Shamanistic medical approaches were freely combined with Western ideas.

The Chinese, Koreans and Japanese have been quite liberal and open-minded about strengthening their medical traditions, by integrating aspects from other cultures. Following the Chinese Cultural Revolution in the mid-twentieth century, the Chinese government took a very active role in integrating Western medicine into its national healthcare system, and made a thorough attempt to modernize traditional Chinese medicine by expunging superstition and conducting rigorous scientific research to investigate the material basis for traditional Eastern medical theories. Today in China, Korea and Japan, one finds a homogeneous, interdisciplinary approach to the practice of medicine, in which Eastern and Western theories are freely intermingled.

Western medical institutions are also beginning to recognize the validity of Eastern medicine, and are incorporating many of its procedures into clinical practice. This is even occurring within the larger HMOs (health maintenance organizations) and health insurance providers, who have been very close-minded to Eastern medicine in the past. There are also many Western healing arts that evolved during the twentieth century that have integrated aspects of both Eastern and Western traditions. They are often labeled as *alternative*, *holistic* or *integrated medicine*.

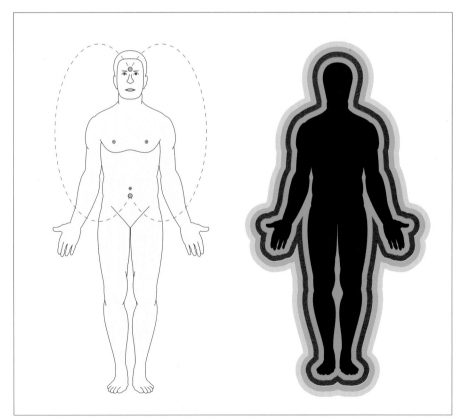

Speculative Eastern concept of human electro-magnetic fields as they relate to Qi energy centers.

Speculative Western concept of the human body as continuous energy fields that form a unified matrix.

Perhaps what we are beginning to see emerge are the first steps toward integrating these different healing traditions into a single, cohesive world view. While this book divides medical concepts into two distinct chapters—Western Concepts and Eastern Concepts—it is important to realize that this distinction is rapidly dissolving in many modern medical practices and colleges, where the emphasis is shifting toward developing a more holistic, scientifically forward-looking medicine.

Emerging Viewpoints
Many modern Western scientists, physicists, and theoreticians have written extensively about bioelectricity, bioenergy and human energy fields. It is now widely understood that the human body produces measurable electromagnetic fields, much like a magnet. This is not surprising in light of the fact that our nervous system essentially communicates via a chain of electrochemical reactions between nerve cells. While most scientists agree on the existence of electromagnetic fields, they are as yet unable to prove the precise role they play in human anatomy and physiology. Many Eastern theoreticians are attempting to correlate human magnetic fields with Eastern meridian theory.

Some progressive thinkers hypothesize that the human body is nothing but energy, and that its physical material form is merely the densest level of energetic matter that exists in a continuous energetic field, emanating outward. Its density is merely what makes it visible and tangible. It is thought that other levels, progressively less energetically dense (hence invisible), surround the physical level. These various levels are suggested in the drawing at left. It is further suggested that this energetic field is organized at the outer level, creating an organizational matrix that eventually builds its way down to the physical level, where it becomes visible and tangible to the human senses. In a sense, this energetic model is the opposite of our current scientific model, which postulates that all energetic organization begins at the molecular level (physical) and builds outward.

Healing and the Martial Arts
Martial artists have always studied the human body for two purposes: to hurt and to heal. This is reflected in the old saying frequently spoken by masters to their students: "Before you learn how to hurt someone, you must first learn how to heal them." Thus, historically, the study of many martial arts began in this dualistic setting, in which the student learned both healing and combative skills. This was particularly true of martial arts that were taught in temples. In many martial arts, this tradition still continues today. To Westerners, this appears contradictory—hurting vs. healing. But to the traditional East Asian mind, complexity, contradiction and ambiguity are the inherent qualities of nature, reflected in the order of the universe.

Today it is widely acknowledged that superiority in martial techniques ultimately comes from an intimate knowledge of the human body. Thus, most contemporary masters of pressure point attacks have extensively studied the foundations of Eastern medicine or related healing arts. This has led them to a superior understanding of the body's weaknesses, allowing them to capitalize on these inherent vulnerabilities. While this knowledge empowers a person with the potential to create greater violence, it also permits one to greatly reduce the level of destruction as well. By manipulating the body's weak points, it becomes possible to immobilize or restrain an attacker without causing serious or permanent injury. One's degree of skill directly influences one's ability to do this safely, without endangering one's self.

It is also important to understand that "combat" is just one aspect of the martial arts, which are also equally concerned with physical well-being and emotional and spiritual evolution. This is what differentiates a "martial art" from a combative system like boxing or wrestling. For the spiritually evolved martial artist, the use of force to resolve a situation always carries with it a social and moral responsibility to apply force in an appropriate and sensible manner.

Simplicity, Faith and Science
Attempting to comprehend the nature of the human body, or the foundations of Western and Eastern medicine, is a daunting task. There are no easy answers or shortcuts to grasping this complex and constantly evolving body of knowledge. As a result, many laypersons gravitate toward practitioners or arts that espouse simplistic viewpoints and easily understood concepts. Sometimes this verges on superstition or blind faith, and is often characterized by a dogmatic adherence to the most traditional and ancient of medical cosmologies. Many martial artists are particularly drawn to simplistic truths, as they are much easier to grasp.

While many of these traditional approaches are often based on concepts that have proven themselves over a 2000 year period, we must be aware that they are nonetheless, 2000 year old concepts. They were the best attempts by the people of that time to understand the workings of the universe and the human body. Naturally, we have learned a great deal since then. Not to consider and integrate this new knowledge is rather foolish, akin to sticking your head in the sand.

While it is tempting to believe that complex concepts can be distilled into simple axioms, it is simply not true—not without sacrificing important content. With respect to Eastern and Western medicine, there are no simple answers, only oversimplifications (a common trend in popular literature). Consequently, this is not a simple book, but rather a book which attempts to simplify *responsibly*, a very complex subject—the essential nature of the human body.

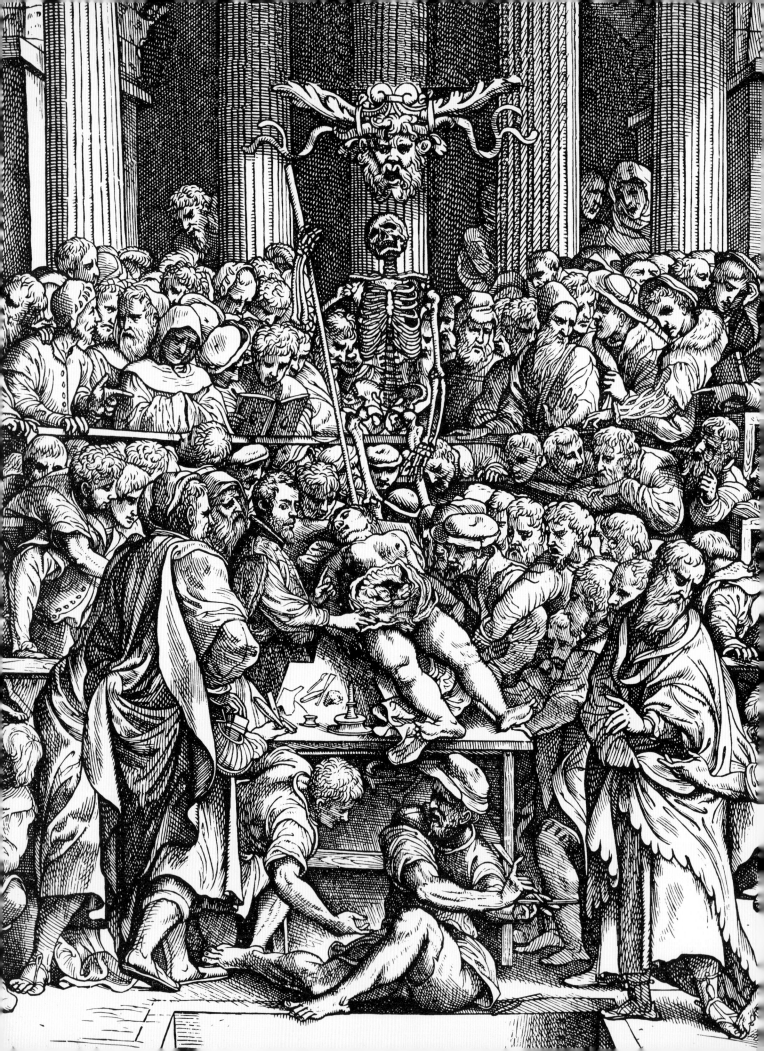

Western medicine traces its modern roots to the ancient Mediterranean world of Plato, Hippocrates and Galen. It is from this tradition that most of the tenets of modern Western medicine arose. Theories of internal structure, pragmatic observation and common sense ideals for dealing with patients all have their birth in this period. Over the centuries, Western medicine continued to evolve according to the spiritual and philosophical traditions of the times, which were largely defined by alchemy, astrology, naturalistic

WESTERN CONCEPTS

concepts and, eventually, powerful Christian religious institutions. Gradually, the rise of secular states and the declining power of the church shifted medicine in the direction of science—a path it has followed ever since. Today Western medicine is widely valued for its ability to treat catastrophic injuries, emergencies and well-defined medical problems, particularly those requiring surgery or the use of high-technology equipment. Often it can define aspects of the body that are imperceptible to Eastern medicine.

Overview

In Western medicine, two branches of learning, human anatomy and physiology, are the cornerstone to understanding the human body. *Human anatomy* is concerned with the study of body structures, and the relationships between those structures. Whereas, *human physiology* deals with how these body structures function to sustain human life. In Western medicine, the combined study of structure (anatomy) and function (physiology) constitutes the basis for understanding the human body. Thus, the structure of a specific body part is believed to determine its functions. For example, the joints of the skull are fused and immobile to protect the brain, whereas the joints of the arm and leg are highly mobile to permit locomotion. Since Western medicine is continually evolving, our understanding of structure and function is constantly expanding and being revised.

Structural Levels

In the Western model, the body consists of multiple levels of *structural organization*, which interact to maintain life. They are:

- Chemical
- Cell
- Tissue
- Organ
- System
- Organism

In a simplistic sense, each of these levels constitute the building blocks leading to a higher level of organization. The process begins at the microscopic level, where chemicals combine to form cells. Cells, in turn, join to form specific tissues, tissues combine to form organs, organs work together in larger systems, and systems function in unison to constitute a total organism—a living human being.

Chemical Level

The chemical level consists of all the chemical substances needed to maintain life. Atoms combine to form molecules, such as proteins, vitamins, carbohydrates and fats.

Cell Level

Cells are created when chemicals combine to form specialized structures that perform specific functions. Muscle cells, nerve cells and blood cells are typical examples.

Tissue Level

Tissues consist of groups of similar cells that perform special functions. For example, a specific type of tissue that lines the stomach, consist of parietal cells that produce hydrochloric acid, mucous cells that secret mucus to protect the stomach lining, and zymogenic cells that produce enzymes to aid digestion.

Organ Level

Organs are structures comprised of two or more different types of tissues. Organs have a distinct shape and perform specific functions. For example, the heart pumps blood and the lungs take in oxygen.

System Level

A system consists of related organs that perform a common function. For example, the digestive system consists of the mouth, throat, stomach, rectum and various other organs, all of which function together to break down and absorb food, and eliminate wastes. Some organs are grouped in more than one system. For example, the pancreas is part of the digestive system and endocrine system.

Organism Level

This is considered the highest level of structural organization, in which all of the body's systems function together to define a living person. Historically, Western medicine has predominantly focused on a *systemic* approach, where diagnosis and treatment focused on the analysis of problems in specific body systems. This is reflected in the many highly specialized branches of medical science that exist, such as neurology. One of the evolving characteristics of progressive, contemporary Western medicine is its increased emphasis on developing a more *organismic*, holistic approach to health and wellness. In this sense, Eastern and Western approaches are becoming more similar.

Principal Body Systems

There are eleven principal systems of the human body, which are shown on the next three pages. For martial artists and practitioners of Eastern healing arts, the most important systems are the skeletal, muscular, nervous and circulatory systems—all of which are outlined in this chapter. Nonetheless, a brief examination of the other systems will lead to a more complete picture. The eleven principal body systems are:

1. Integumentary

This system comprises the skin and structures stemming from it—hair, nails, oil glands and sweat glands. Its functions are to regulate body temperature, protect the body, eliminate wastes, and receive specific stimuli (e.g., temperature, pressure and pain).

2. Skeletal

This system comprises all of the body's bones, cartilages and joints. Its functions are to support and protect the body, assist locomotion, produce blood cells and store minerals.

3. Muscular

This system comprises all of the body's muscle tissue. Its functions are to initiate movement, maintain posture and produce heat.

4. Circulatory

This system consists of the heart, blood and blood vessels. Its functions are to distribute oxygen and nutrients, remove wastes, and regulate pH, body temperature, and the water content of cells.

5. Lymphatic / Immunologic

This systems consists of lymph, lymphatic vessels, and organs containing lymphatic tissue, such as the spleen and tonsils. Its functions are to transport proteins, plasma and fats; filter body fluid; produce white blood cells; and defend against disease.

6. Nervous

This system consists of the brain, spinal cord, nerves, and sense organs such as the eyes. Its functions are to control and integrate body activities by sending nerve impulses.

7. Endocrine

This system consists of glands and tissues that produce hormones. Its functions are to control and integrate body activities by sending chemical signals (hormones) via the blood.

8. Respiratory

This system consists of the lungs and related passageways, such as the throat (pharynx), windpipe (trachea), voice box (larynx) and bronchial tubes. Its functions are to supply oxygen, remove carbon dioxide, and regulate the body's pH balance.

9. Digestive

This system consists of a long tube called the gastrointestinal tract, and related organs such as the mouth, salivary glands, liver, gallbladder and pancreas. Its functions are to break down and absorb food, and eliminate wastes.

10. Urinary

This system consists of organs such as the kidneys, ureters, urinary bladder and urethra. Its functions are to eliminate wastes, and regulate blood chemistry, red blood cell count, pH balance, fluid volume, and electrolyte balance.

11. Reproductive

This system consists of organs that produce, transport or store reproductive cells. Its function is to reproduce the human species.

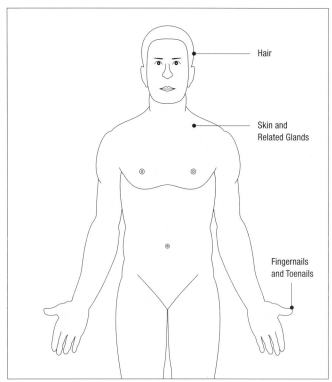

Hair

Skin and Related Glands

Fingernails and Toenails

1. Integumentary System

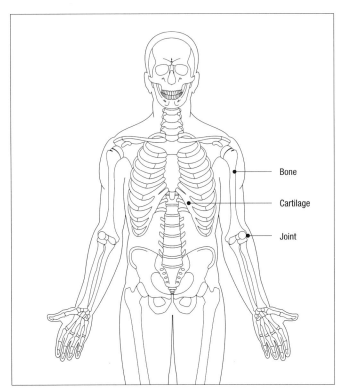

Bone

Cartilage

Joint

2. Skeletal System

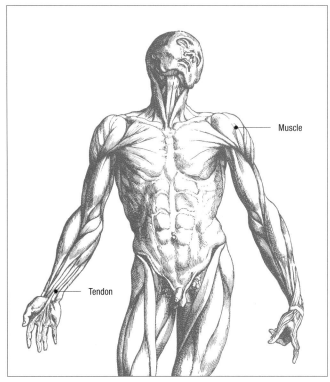

Muscle

Tendon

3. Muscular System

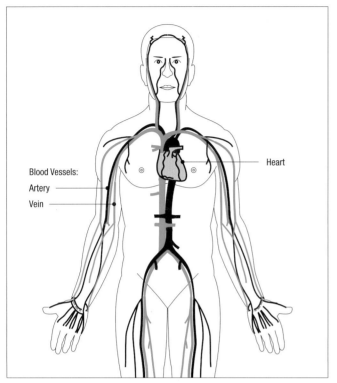

4. *Circulatory System*

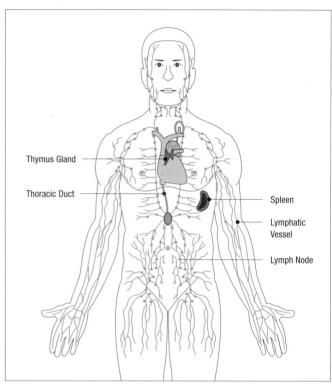

5. *Lymphatic / Immunologic System*

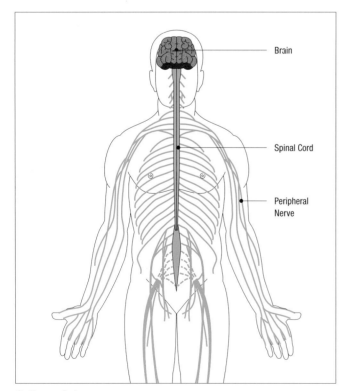

6. *Nervous System*

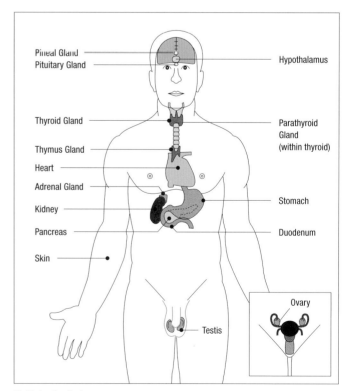

7. *Endocrine System*

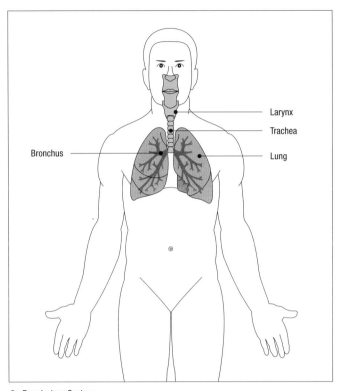

Larynx

Trachea

Bronchus

Lung

8. Respiratory System

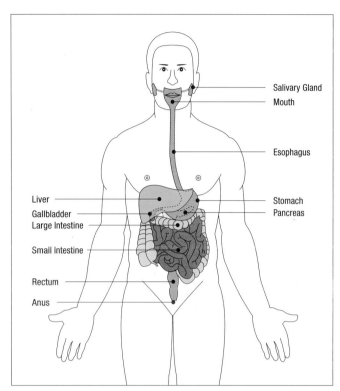

Salivary Gland

Mouth

Esophagus

Liver

Gallbladder

Large Intestine

Small Intestine

Stomach

Pancreas

Rectum

Anus

9. Digestive System

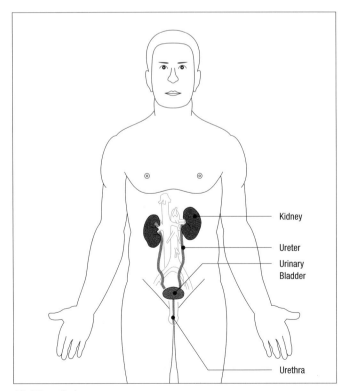

Kidney

Ureter

Urinary Bladder

Urethra

10. Urinary System

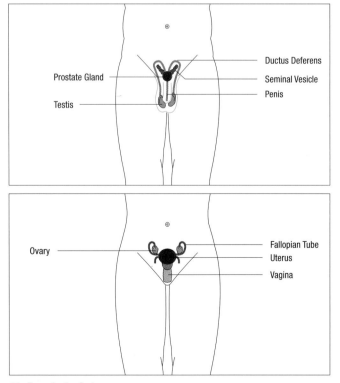

Prostate Gland

Testis

Ductus Deferens

Seminal Vesicle

Penis

Ovary

Fallopian Tube

Uterus

Vagina

11. Reproductive System

The human body consists of approximately 206 separate skeletal bones, which in conjunction with muscles and tissue, provide the framework that allows a human being to stand upright and move. The bones are joined to each other by movable connections called joints. From a martial artist's point of view, these joints are weak points to be exploited (on others) or protected (on yourself). Bone joints vary widely in terms of structure, strength and function. Joints found in the arms and legs are highly mobile, as would be expected. The joints of the spinal column are much less so, since they must also protect major nerves that pass through the vertebrae. The joints linking the bones of the skull together (called sutures) are totally immobile, except during infancy.

Bones are composed primarily of calcium phosphate, which contributes hardness, and collagen, the body's supporting tissue. The bones are wrapped in a membrane (called periosteum) containing blood vessels and nerve fibers. Bone is living tissue and is constantly renewing and reforming itself. Constant muscular activity strengthens bone by causing the bone to adapt and reform along the lines of stress. For martial artists, dietary calcium is important for maintaining bone strength, particularly for women, in whom calcium loss accelerates rapidly after age forty. Basic bone injuries are as follows:

Bone Bruise

A strong blow to the bone can cause damage to surface tissue, leading to bleeding under the periosteum. The heel, forearm, shin and knuckle are the bones most frequently bruised as a result of striking, blocking, being hit, or landing incorrectly when jumping or falling. Bone bruises to the knuckles are common when breaking boards or bricks, or continually striking hard surfaces. Bones that are repeatedly bruised tend to form additional bone in the damaged area, which can lead to an increase in overall bone mass.

Periostitis

Periostitis is an inflammation of the periosteum caused by overuse and often precedes a stress fracture. Shin splints are a typical example. Rest is needed to allow the bone to heal and avoid a stress fracture.

*Note:
The *Xiphoid Process,* attached to the sternum at one end, consists of cartilage which changes to bone as we age, fully hardening at about forty. When striking or pressing this area on older individuals, the Xiphoid Process may fracture, separating from the sternum and driving into the liver. Do not strike this area during martial arts training.

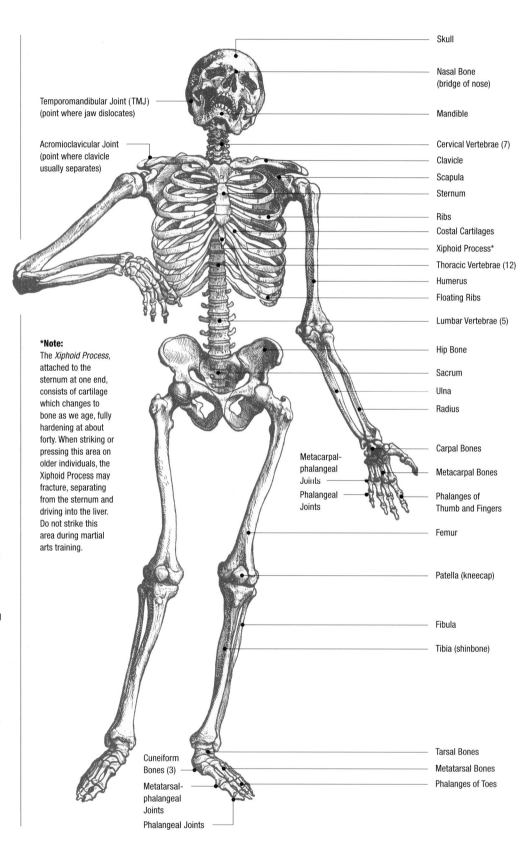

Temporomandibular Joint (TMJ)
(point where jaw dislocates)

Acromioclavicular Joint
(point where clavicle usually separates)

Skull

Nasal Bone
(bridge of nose)

Mandible

Cervical Vertebrae (7)

Clavicle

Scapula

Sternum

Ribs

Costal Cartilages

Xiphoid Process*

Thoracic Vertebrae (12)

Humerus

Floating Ribs

Lumbar Vertebrae (5)

Hip Bone

Sacrum

Ulna

Radius

Metacarpal-phalangeal Joints

Phalangeal Joints

Carpal Bones

Metacarpal Bones

Phalanges of Thumb and Fingers

Femur

Patella (kneecap)

Fibula

Tibia (shinbone)

Cuneiform Bones (3)

Metatarsal-phalangeal Joints

Phalangeal Joints

Tarsal Bones

Metatarsal Bones

Phalanges of Toes

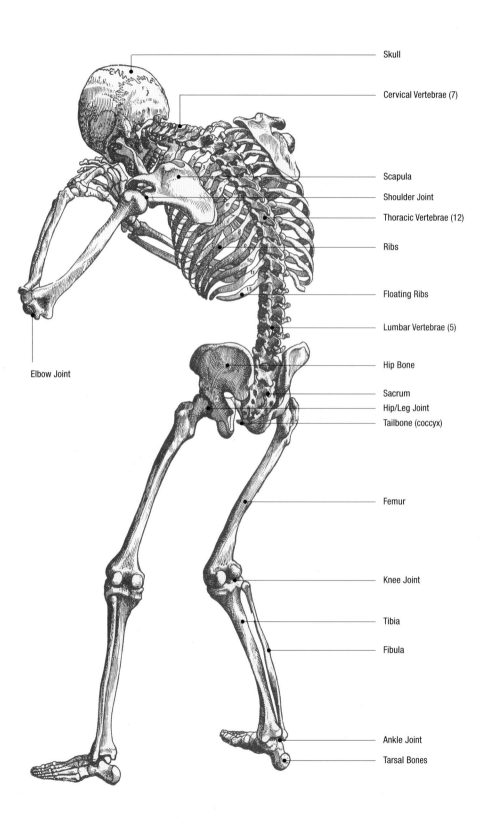

Skull

Cervical Vertebrae (7)

Scapula
Shoulder Joint
Thoracic Vertebrae (12)
Ribs

Floating Ribs

Lumbar Vertebrae (5)

Hip Bone

Sacrum
Hip/Leg Joint
Tailbone (coccyx)

Femur

Knee Joint

Tibia
Fibula

Ankle Joint
Tarsal Bones

Elbow Joint

Stress Fracture

Stress fractures are small breaks in the surface of the bone, usually caused by over-use. Injuries to the feet and shin (tibia) are more common, particularly among women, who tend to have less bone mass. Injuries to the femoral neck and pelvis can also occur.

Fracture

Fractures are cracks or separations of the bone, and are usually caused by stress or a blow. They normally bring immediate and severe pain and are often the result of a trauma sustained when striking, blocking, being hit, or falling improperly. There are three grades of fractures: *closed* (crack), *open* (bone protrudes from beneath skin), and *comminuted* (broken in more than one place). Serious fractures may also involve nerve damage.

Dislocation

When a joint is twisted, hyperextended, or struck with a hard blow, it will move out of normal alignment, often damaging supporting ligaments, cartilage, tendons, nerves and blood vessels. Bone chips may be present. Thumb, hip, shoulder and spinal dislocations are considered serious injuries. Untrained efforts to reset a dislocation can cause nerve, bone and joint damage.

Joint Breaking Force

The list below gives the relative force required to break or separate joints or bones. The actual force required will vary based on individual anatomy and method of stress.

Skull (at temple)	moderate
Nasal Bone (downward blow)	moderate
Clavicle at shoulder (separation)	moderate
Shoulder (dislocation)	high
Elbow Joint	moderate
Wrist Joint	moderate
Finger Joints	very low
Thumb Joints	low
Cervical Spine	moderate
Thoracic/Lumbar Spine	high
Hip Joints, Hip Bone	very high
Kneecap (lateral dislocation)	moderate
Knee Joint (break)	high
Ankle Joint	high
Big Toe Joints	low
Small Toe Joints	very low

The muscular system consists of about 700 *skeletal muscles* which attach to bones, forming our basic method of mobility. The bones act as levers, the joints as fulcrums, the muscles move these structures to produce movement when triggered by a nerve impulse. Muscles also assist in blood circulation and protect and confine organs.

Skeletal muscles are attached to bones by dense, white, fibrous cords called tendons. Muscles produce movement by exerting force on tendons, which then pull bones or other structures such as skin. Muscles that contract rapidly are primarily used for speed. Their fibers usually run parallel to one another and converge on a central tendon, such as the gastrocnemius muscle on the calf. Muscles that contract more slowly are primarily used for power. Their fibers often converge from all directions on the tendon, such as the deltoid muscle on the shoulder. Basically, two types of muscle fibers are found in all muscles: slow-twitch fibers (which contract slowly) and fast-twitch fibers (which contract more rapidly). It is believed that the ratio of slow-twitch to fast-twitch fibers, which is genetically determined, determines overall muscle speed and power. Athletes with superior speed have been found to contain higher percentages of fast-twitch fibers, while athletes with greater endurance have more slow-twitch fibers. The drawings at right show major *superficial muscles,* located near the body's surface.

Muscle Damage

Damage to muscle tissue impairs mobility and reduces circulation. A direct blow or twisting hold can damage blood vessels in the muscle, causing internal bleeding, blood clotting and spasms. Muscle and tendon *strains* are defined as a tear in the surface and may be quite painful. A more serious *rupture* is defined as a partial or complete separation of the connections between muscle, tendon or bone. This usually results in extreme pain and muscle spasms, making movement difficult or impossible. Strains and ruptures can also be caused by excessive muscle stress, overuse, or failure to warm-up properly. Scar tissue, which forms after a muscle injury, is more susceptible to damage, particularly as we become older.

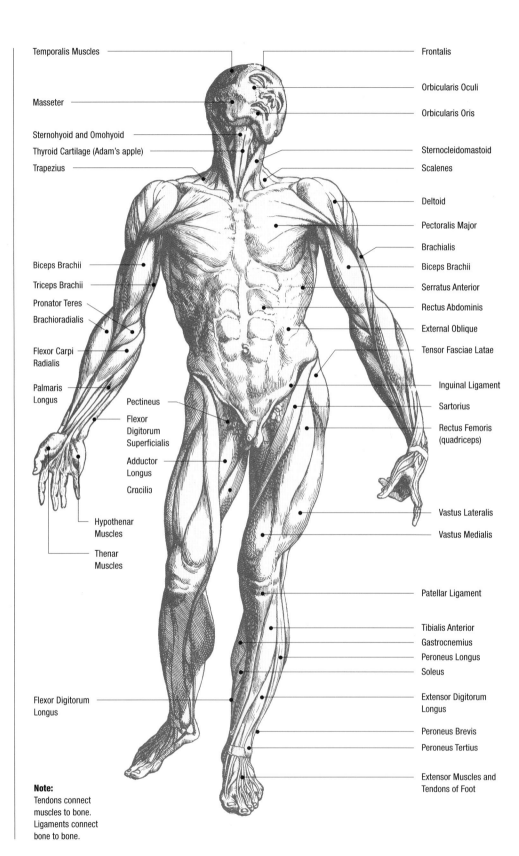

Temporalis Muscles

Masseter

Sternohyoid and Omohyoid

Thyroid Cartilage (Adam's apple)

Trapezius

Biceps Brachii

Triceps Brachii

Pronator Teres

Brachioradialis

Flexor Carpi Radialis

Palmaris Longus

Pectineus

Flexor Digitorum Superficialis

Adductor Longus

Gracilis

Hypothenar Muscles

Thenar Muscles

Flexor Digitorum Longus

Frontalis

Orbicularis Oculi

Orbicularis Oris

Sternocleidomastoid

Scalenes

Deltoid

Pectoralis Major

Brachialis

Biceps Brachii

Serratus Anterior

Rectus Abdominis

External Oblique

Tensor Fasciae Latae

Inguinal Ligament

Sartorius

Rectus Femoris (quadriceps)

Vastus Lateralis

Vastus Medialis

Patellar Ligament

Tibialis Anterior

Gastrocnemius

Peroneus Longus

Soleus

Extensor Digitorum Longus

Peroneus Brevis

Peroneus Tertius

Extensor Muscles and Tendons of Foot

Note:
Tendons connect muscles to bone. Ligaments connect bone to bone.

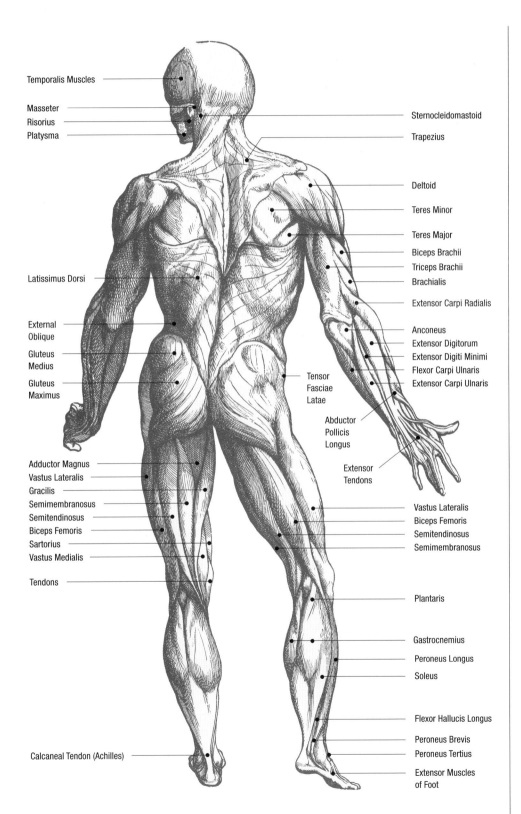

Temporalis Muscles

Masseter
Risorius
Platysma

Sternocleidomastoid

Trapezius

Deltoid

Teres Minor

Teres Major
Biceps Brachii
Triceps Brachii
Brachialis

Extensor Carpi Radialis

Anconeus
Extensor Digitorum
Extensor Digiti Minimi
Flexor Carpi Ulnaris
Extensor Carpi Ulnaris

Latissimus Dorsi

External
Oblique

Gluteus
Medius

Gluteus
Maximus

Tensor
Fasciae
Latae

Abductor
Pollicis
Longus

Extensor
Tendons

Adductor Magnus
Vastus Lateralis
Gracilis
Semimembranosus
Semitendinosus
Biceps Femoris
Sartorius
Vastus Medialis

Tendons

Vastus Lateralis
Biceps Femoris
Semitendinosus
Semimembranosus

Plantaris

Gastrocnemius
Peroneus Longus
Soleus

Flexor Hallucis Longus

Peroneus Brevis
Peroneus Tertius

Extensor Muscles
of Foot

Calcaneal Tendon (Achilles)

Muscle Nomenclature

The names of skeletal muscles are derived from Latin terms that define specific characteristics, such as direction of muscle fibers, location, size, shape, number of origins, places of origin, and type of action. Common terms are listed below.

Direction

Rectus: Parallel to body midline
Transverse: Perpendicular to body midline
Oblique: Diagonal to body midline
("midline" denotes the body's vertical axis)

Location

Terms designating location are taken from the names of close structures. (e.g., the temporalis muscle is near the temporal bone.)

Size

Maximus: Largest
Minimus: Smallest
Longus: Long
Brevis: Short

Shape

Deltoid: Triangular shape
Trapezius: Trapezoid shape
Serratus: Saw-toothed shape
Rhomboid: Diamond shape

Number of Origins

Biceps: Two-headed muscle (2 origins)
Triceps: Three-headed muscle (3 origins)
Quadriceps: Four-headed muscle (4 origins)

Place of Origin and Insertion

Terms are taken from the names of structures. For example, the sternocleidomastoid muscle originates on the sternum and clavicle, and inserts at the mastoid process.

Type of Action

Flexor: Decreases joint angle
Extensor: Increases joint angle
Abductor: Moves bone away from midline
Adductor: Moves bone closer to midline
Levator: Produces upward movement
Depressor: Produces downward movement
Supinator: Palm turns up or anteriorly
Pronator: Palm turns down or posteriorly
Sphincter: Decreases size of an opening
Tensor: Produces rigidity in a body part
Rotator: Moves bone around long axis

The nervous system is one of the body's crucial control and integrating centers. While it has been extensively studied by Western medicine for centuries, it remains relatively poorly understood when compared to other body systems. In traditional Eastern medicine, the concept is non-existent.

The nervous system helps control and integrate all of the body's activities, internally and externally, by sensing changes and then interpreting and reacting to them. Its most important components are the brain and the spinal cord. *Cranial nerves* emerging from the brain, and *spinal nerves* emerging from the spinal cord, distribute themselves throughout the body in a vast, complex network integrating all of the body's functions (muscular, neurological, glandular, etc.). Nerve impulses, defined as tiny electrochemical currents, travel along nerves to communicate between the brain, muscles, skin, organs, glands, blood vessels, and other parts of the body. The preceding description is a vast simplification of very complex subject. However, further discussion is not particularly relevant to martial artists' needs.

Martial artists primarily study the nervous system to better understand how to control, damage, or heal the human body. Nerve attacks are used to generate pain, cause involuntary muscle responses, or impair motor functions. When we generate pain in another person, we encourage that person to do something they would not otherwise do (retreat, submit, enter a hold, release a hold, fall down, etc.).

The location of specific nerves (as identified by Western medicine) often corresponds to the position of specific acupoints (as identified by Eastern medicine). Locations of acupoints, cross referenced to nerves, are outlined later under *Meridian Reference*. Remember, the system you use (nerves vs. acupoints) is not nearly as important as knowing pressure point locations, what they affect, and how to achieve consistent results. The illustration at right shows the major nerve plexuses (networks) and branches, as viewed from the front and back. Points sensitive to pressure may involve many other minor nerves or combinations of nerves.

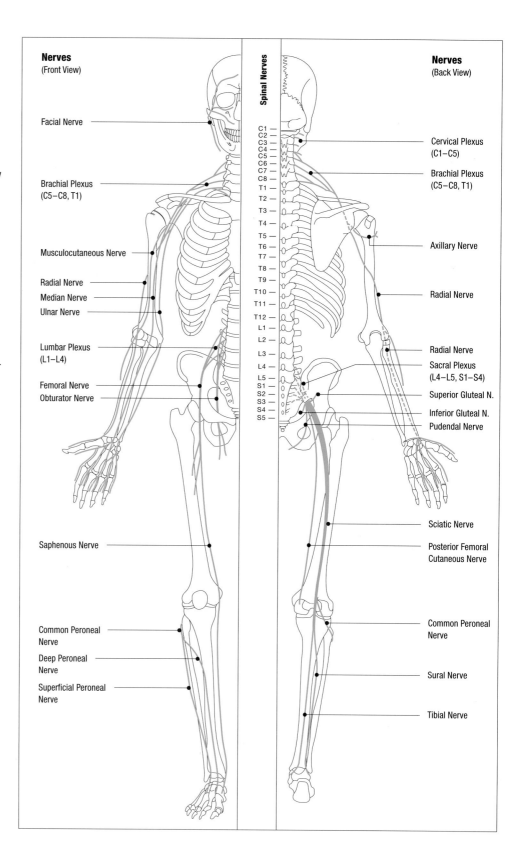

Nerves (Front View)

Facial Nerve

Brachial Plexus (C5–C8, T1)

Musculocutaneous Nerve

Radial Nerve

Median Nerve

Ulnar Nerve

Lumbar Plexus (L1–L4)

Femoral Nerve

Obturator Nerve

Saphenous Nerve

Common Peroneal Nerve

Deep Peroneal Nerve

Superficial Peroneal Nerve

Spinal Nerves

C1
C2
C3
C4
C5
C6
C7
C8
T1
T2
T3
T4
T5
T6
T7
T8
T9
T10
T11
T12
L1
L2
L3
L4
L5
S1
S2
S3
S4
S5

Nerves (Back View)

Cervical Plexus (C1–C5)

Brachial Plexus (C5–C8, T1)

Axillary Nerve

Radial Nerve

Radial Nerve

Sacral Plexus (L4–L5, S1–S4)

Superior Gluteal N.

Inferior Gluteal N.

Pudendal Nerve

Sciatic Nerve

Posterior Femoral Cutaneous Nerve

Common Peroneal Nerve

Sural Nerve

Tibial Nerve

Distribution of Spinal Nerves to Dermatomes

Each spinal nerve supplies a localized area of skin as shown. In actuality, dermatomes edges are not clearly defined, but overlap with adjacent areas. Dermatomes also vary individually.

C – Cervical
T – Thoracic
L – Lumber
S – Sacral

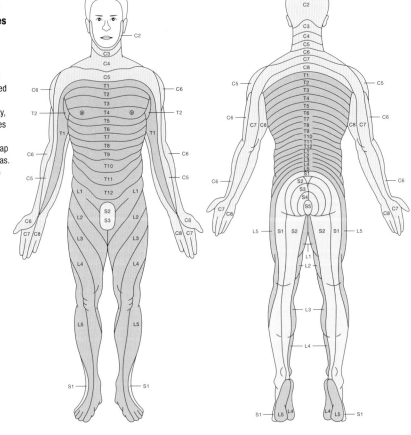

Major Nerves

Cranial Nerves
Twelve pairs of nerves (identified by Roman numerals and names) leave the brain, pass through the skull, and supply the head, neck, and part of the trunk.

Olfactory Nerve (I)
Optic Nerve (II)
Oculomotor Nerve (III)
Trochlear Nerve (IV)
Trigeminal Nerve (V)
Abducent Nerve (VI)
Facial Nerve (VII)
Vestibulocochlear Nerve (VIII)
Glossopharyngeal Nerve (IX)
Vagus Nerve (X)
Accessory Nerve (XI)
Hypoglossal Nerve (XII)

Cervical Plexus (C1–C5)
Supplies the skin and muscles of head, neck, and upper shoulders; connects with cranial nerves XI and XII; supplies the diaphragm (breathing functions).

Lesser Occipital Nerve C2
Great Auricular Nerve C2, C3
Transverse Cervical Nerve C2, C3
Supraclavicular Nerve C3, C4
Phrenic Nerve (to diaphragm) C3–C5

Brachial Plexus (C5–C8, T1)
Supplies the upper extremities and numerous neck and shoulder muscles.

Musculocutaneous Nerve C5–C7
Median Nerve C5–C8, T1
Axillary Nerve C7, C8, T1
Radial Nerve C5–C8, T1
Ulnar Nerve C7, C8, T1

Thoracic Nerves (T1–T12)
Supplies the trunk primarily; and connects with some nerves in the brachial plexus.

Lumbar Plexus (L1–L4)
Supplies the abdominal wall (front and side), external genitals, and part of the lower extremities.

Iliohypogastric Nerve L1
Ilio-inguinal Nerve L1
Genitofemoral Nerve L1, L2
Lateral Femoral Cutaneous Nerve L2, L3
Femoral Nerve L2–L4
Obturator Nerve L2–L4

Sacral Plexus (L4–L5, S1–S4)
Supplies the buttocks, perineum (space between anus and genitalia), and lower extremities. The sciatic nerve (the largest nerve in the body) supplies the entire musculature of the leg and foot.

Superior Gluteal Nerve L4, L5, S1
Inferior Gluteal Nerve L5, S1, S2
Common Peroneal Nerve L4, L5, S1, S2
Posterior Femoral Cutaneous Nerve S2, S3
Sciatic Nerve L4, L5, S1–S3
Tibial Nerve L4, L5, S1–S3
Pudendal Nerve S2–S4

Spinal Nerves and Branches
The spine consists of numerous individual bony structures (vertebrae) connected to each other by fibrous shock absorbers (intervertebral discs). At the base of the spine is the tailbone (coccyx), which serves no function but is very painful when struck. The *spinal nerves* (31 pairs) emerge from the spinal cord at each intervertebral disc and are identified with alphanumeric names (see illustration on preceding page). Each nerve supplies a specific part of the body. All spinal nerves (except T2–T11) form nerve networks called plexuses, from which nerves emerge serving specific regions. The T2–T11 nerves (called thoracic nerves) do not form plexuses but channel directly to the areas they supply.

Attacks to the spinal nerves (at the neck or along the back) will damage the nerve supply to specific areas. For example, a blow to the head or neck causing compression of the C6 and C7 nerve roots in the spine may produce pain or numbness, or impair muscle functions along the back of shoulder, elbow, or all the way out to the hand (depending on the location and severity of the blow).

In Western medicine, skin sensation is mapped out in defined areas called *dermatomes*. Each area corresponds to a specific spinal nerve root. Dermatomes are normally used to diagnose nerve problems, but can also be used by martial artists to verify nerve locations by cross-reference with tables listing nerves and their origin. For example, if you press or hit the ulnar nerve at the back of the elbow, one should feel numbness or a tingling sensation in the vicinity of the fourth and fifth fingers (C8 dermatome).

Nerve Damage
Damage to nerves from blows or pressure can result in pain, numbness, or paralysis; problems using muscles or moving certain appendages; problems with organs; or inability to sense certain stimuli (taste, touch, vision, smell, sound). Symptoms can be permanent or transient, taking months or years to disappear. Some nerves repair themselves, others do not. Severe damage to spinal nerves is believed to be permanent, as they do not appear to regenerate. Medical opinion in this area is evolving.

The continual circulation of blood is essential to human life. Blood transports oxygen, nutrients and hormones, and removes carbon dioxide and other wastes, sustaining millions of individual cells found throughout the body. Blood also regulates pH, body temperature and the water content of cells.

The blood circulates in the following manner. Blood is pumped from the right side of the heart into the lungs, where oxygen diffuses into the bloodstream. The blood continues to the left side of the heart, and is then pumped out to organs, muscles and cells through a network of blood vessels called arteries, arterioles and capillaries. Arteries carry blood from the heart to various parts of the body, branching into smaller vessels called arterioles, which branch into a network of microscopic vessels called capillaries. Capillaries allow the exchange of vital materials between blood and tissue cells. The blood returns to the heart by draining from the capillaries into tiny vessels called venules, which merge into larger vessels called veins, eventually flowing into the heart where it is recirculated.

Major blood vessels often align with major nerves and are sometimes closely related to the positions of acupoint meridians in Eastern medicine. The illustrations at right show the major blood vessels.

Interrupting Circulation

Martial artists study the location of major blood vessels in order to make more efficient attacks, as well as to better protect their own vulnerable areas. In martial arts, normal blood circulation may be interrupted by applying chokes to the carotid artery on the neck (cutting off oxygen to the brain), by striking the chest (causing the heart to beat irregularly or stop altogether), by cutting or puncturing vital areas with a sharp weapon (causing external blood loss), or by striking vital areas (causing internal bleeding). A proper choke at the carotid artery causes complete interruption of the blood supply, leading to loss of consciousness in about 15 seconds (a poor choke takes longer, since partial blood-flow is present). Chokes can also lead to stoppage of breathing and/or cardiac arrest. Failure to restore normal

Arteries

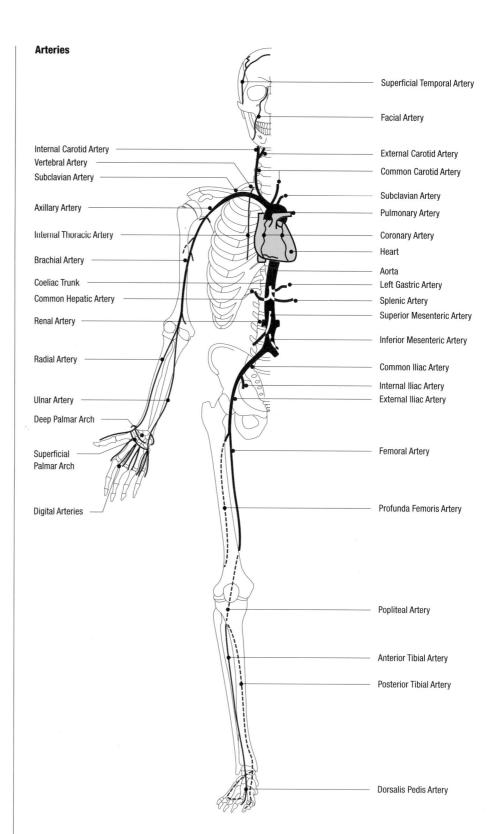

Superficial Temporal Artery

Facial Artery

Internal Carotid Artery

Vertebral Artery

Subclavian Artery

External Carotid Artery

Common Carotid Artery

Axillary Artery

Subclavian Artery

Pulmonary Artery

Internal Thoracic Artery

Coronary Artery

Brachial Artery

Heart

Coeliac Trunk

Aorta

Common Hepatic Artery

Left Gastric Artery

Splenic Artery

Renal Artery

Superior Mesenteric Artery

Inferior Mesenteric Artery

Radial Artery

Common Iliac Artery

Internal Iliac Artery

Ulnar Artery

External Iliac Artery

Deep Palmar Arch

Superficial
Palmar Arch

Femoral Artery

Digital Arteries

Profunda Femoris Artery

Popliteal Artery

Anterior Tibial Artery

Posterior Tibial Artery

Dorsalis Pedis Artery

Veins

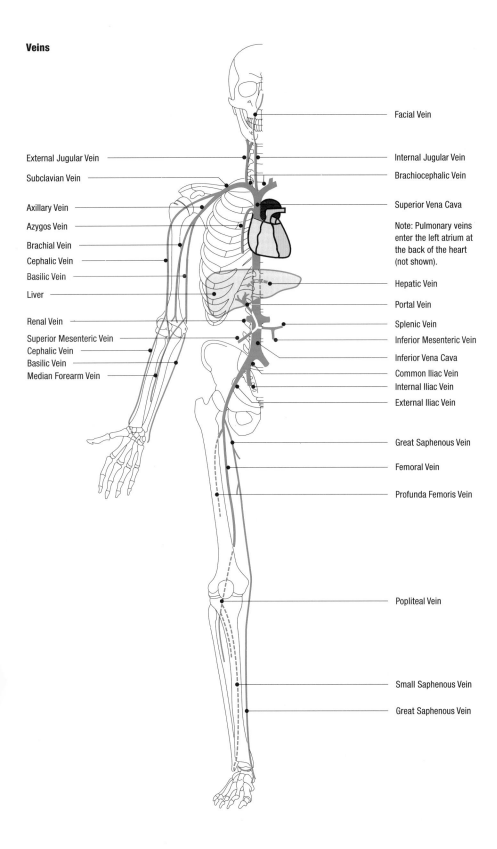

External Jugular Vein

Subclavian Vein

Axillary Vein

Azygos Vein

Brachial Vein

Cephalic Vein

Basilic Vein

Liver

Renal Vein

Superior Mesenteric Vein

Cephalic Vein

Basilic Vein

Median Forearm Vein

Facial Vein

Internal Jugular Vein

Brachiocephalic Vein

Superior Vena Cava

Note: Pulmonary veins enter the left atrium at the back of the heart (not shown).

Hepatic Vein

Portal Vein

Splenic Vein

Inferior Mesenteric Vein

Inferior Vena Cava

Common Iliac Vein

Internal Iliac Vein

External Iliac Vein

Great Saphenous Vein

Femoral Vein

Profunda Femoris Vein

Popliteal Vein

Small Saphenous Vein

Great Saphenous Vein

breathing and blood circulation results in progressive brain damage and eventually death in a manner of minutes. *Do not* practice chokes, except under the qualified supervision of persons experienced in revival techniques. All vascular chokes result in loss of oxygen to the brain, which destroys brain cells. It is believed that this type of brain damage is permanent and cumulative. Thus, use common sense when training. Most medical experts agree that "being repeatedly choked-out," is not a healthy activity.

Blood Loss

Major blood vessels are most susceptible to slashing attacks from weapons such as knives, at locations where vessels are close to the body's surface. Vital targets include the front of the neck (carotid artery, jugular vein); the side of the jaw (facial artery and vein); the inside of the upper arm near the armpit (brachial artery); the inner wrist (radial and ulnar arteries); the back of the hand (various arteries and veins); the inside of the knee around the joint (great saphenous vein, branches of femoral artery); and the top of the foot (dorsalis pedis artery and vein).

The average adult male contains 5–6 liters of blood (female 4–5). Blood loss greater than 30% results in progressive weakness, shock, profound depression of body processes, coma, and eventually death. Bleeding from arteries causes the fastest loss of blood, since these vessels are connected to the output side of the heart. Arterial bleeding is usually characterized by a pulsing or spurting of bright red blood and can be fatal in as little as a few minutes if not stopped. Venous bleeding is usually dark red and flows smoothly, without spurting. After significant blood loss, red blood cell count and hemo-globin may return to normal in 4–6 weeks.

Effects of Aging

General cardiovascular changes associated with aging include size reduction in heart muscle fiber, loss of heart muscle strength, reduced blood output from the heart, a decline in maximum heart rate, and an increase in systolic blood pressure. By age 80, cerebral blood flow is 20 percent less, and renal blood flow is 50 percent less than in the same individual at age 30.

修真圖

The martial and healing arts of the Far East have a long, rich and intertwined tradition that is intimately associated with the cultures of China, Korea and Japan. Over the millennia, these cultures gave rise to many innovative spiritual and philosophical traditions, which served as the foundation for evolving their own unique healing traditions—the most notable being Chinese medicine. These traditions gradually merged with one another, assimilated Western medical concepts and technologies, and evolved

EASTERN CONCEPTS

into eclectic, homogeneous systems of integrated medicine, espousing a holistic approach to health and wellness. Today there are many different types of healing arts being practiced under the umbrella term, "Eastern medicine." They can involve anything from modern biomedicine to ancient shamanistic rituals. Above all, however, Eastern medicine is widely valued for its holistic, preventative-oriented emphasis and its ability to treat a wide range of illnesses for which Western medicine has no immediate answers.

This chapter will provide an introduction to Eastern concepts of the body as postulated by Eastern medicine in general, and Chinese medicine in particular. The Chinese system has become the most widely documented and practiced among Eastern systems, particularly in the Western world. It is also the system from which most other East Asian systems emerged, and will be the basis for information presented in this section.

Overview

Eastern medicine embodies a holistic approach in which the body is viewed as a single, integrated system, intimately linked to the surrounding universe. A complex network of *meridians* distributes *Qi* (vital energy) throughout the body, vitalizing cells, tissue, organs and other body systems. The health of the body's parts is dependent on the wellness of the whole. Alternating states of health or illness are defined as resulting from a balance, imbalance or disruption in one's Qi.

The sensitive points used in Eastern medicine to manipulate Qi-flow are called *acupoints.* They are the points where the Qi-flow comes to the body's surface, and have been defined as points of high electrical conductivity, acting as amplifiers for Qi flowing along meridians. Qi-flow can be manipulated at acupoints by physical intervention (needles, fingertip pressure, suction), thermal stimulation (burning herbs on or above skin; called moxibustion), and electrical stimulation (below, on or above skin). Qi-flow can also affected by ingested substances (herbs, drugs), meditation, or movement (yoga, Qigong, Tai Chi Chuan, etc.).

BASIC PRINCIPLES

Traditional Eastern medicine evolved over a period of more than 3000 years, and was also heavily influenced by the philosophical and religious traditions of the cultures from which it developed. It is virtually impossible to grasp the nature of Eastern medicine, or practice it competently, without some understanding of its philosophical underpinnings. While it is beyond the scope of this book to present these concepts in any detail, several

important ideas will be outlined in brief, before preceding to a more detailed presentation of Eastern concepts of the human body.

Yin and Yang

The East Asian concept of "yin and yang" postulates that all transformation occurs by the constant interplay of two universal primal states of being. They were first called *the firm* and *the yielding,* and later expressed as *yang* and *yin* (*yo* and *in* in Japanese, *yang* and *um* in Korean). Yang, the firm (depicted by an unbroken line ——), and Yin, the yielding (depicted by a broken line – –), symbolize the two great forces at play in the universe. These forces exist in all things, in a state of constant tension and balance. One defines the other and each contains within it the seed of its opposite; one in essence but two in manifestation, always in flux. In Eastern thought, yin-yang forces of change can be seen operating in natural cycles such as day and night, winter and summer. Typical correspondences are listed at lower-right. In traditional Eastern medicine, yin-yang correspondences form the basis of diagnosis and treatment.

The yin-yang symbol, called the *Tai Chi* (meaning "supreme ultimate"), depicts the two great forces in perfect balance and perpetual alteration, with yang becoming yin, and yin becoming yang; each possessing within itself the embryo of the other. This well known symbol represents the perfection of balance and harmony, and the creative union of opposites throughout the universe. It is widely represented throughout Asian art and culture and is even incorporated into national symbols, such as the South Korean flag.

The illustration at lower-left shows the Tai Chi, surrounded by the eight trigrams symbolizing the primary combinations of yin and yang forces (the numbers have been added and correspond to the key below the drawing). These trigrams were conceived as symbols of all that happens in heaven and on earth, and represent the nature of changing transitional states. Each trigram consists of a unique combination of yin and yang lines, and are classified as described in the illustration. These ideas are outlined further in the 3000 year old Chinese classic text, the *I Ching.*

Tai Chi Symbol + Trigrams

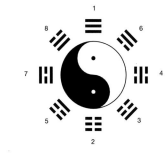

	Trigram Name	Attribute	Image
1	the Creative	strong	heaven
2	the Receptive	yielding	earth
3	the Arousing	movement	thunder
4	the Abysmal	dangerous	water
5	Keeping Still	resting	mountain
6	the Gentle	penetrating	wind, wood
7	the Clinging	light-giving	fire
8	the Joyous	joyful	lake

Yin-Yang Correspondences

Yin	Yang
Earth	Heaven
Female	Male
Night	Day
Moon	Sun
Low	High
Heaviness	Lightness
Falling Tendency	Rising Tendency
Movement inward	Movement outward
Relative stasis	Clear action
Interior	Exterior
Front	Back
Lower section	Upper section
Bones	Skin
Inner organs	Outer organs
Blood	Qi
Inhibition	Stimulation
Deficiency	Excess
Yielding	Firm
Essence	Spirit

The Five Phases

In ancient Chinese thought, Qi was said to give the world substance through its manifestation in the *five phases* of the universe—wood, fire earth, metal and water. This concept is believed to have evolved around 400 BC and to have subsequently spread throughout neighboring regions.

The five phases represent the *process of change,* and were an attempt by ancient minds to understand the workings of the universe. The ancient Chinese used the five phases to develop a system of *cyclical patterns* and *correspondences,* within which all natural phenomena are organized in ways that relate to the process of change. Each of the five phases symbolizes a grouping of related qualities and functions. In the West, the five phases are also commonly called the *five elements*, which has led many people to incorrectly assume that the five phases are elemental materials from which all things are created.

In time, the five phases became the basis for classifying all known natural phenomena, including emotions, colors, sounds, tastes, odors, animals, plants, political structures, weather and planets. The five phases were also related to the human body by traditional Eastern medicine, which discovered phase relationships with organs and anatomical regions. The table at lower-right shows typical correspondences.

The five phases can be sequentially ordered into thirty-six possible cyclical patterns. The two patterns most important to traditional Eastern medicine and the martial arts are called the *production cycle* (also called creation cycle) and the *conquest cycle* (also called destruction cycle). They are used extensively in traditional Eastern medical diagnosis, pathology, and treatment, and to select acupoints for healing. Martial artists often apply the same theories when selecting acupoint targets for fighting. This is covered in detail in the *Martial Applications* chapter, under *Pressure Point Fighting.*

In the *production cycle,* wood produces fire, fire produces earth, earth produces metal, metal produces water, water produces wood, beginning the cycle again. In the *conquest cycle,* wood conquers earth, earth conquers water, water conquers fire, fire conquers metal, metal conquers wood, etc. These two basic cycles are depicted at top-right.

The global view underlying the five phase theory, "a system of correspondences," forms the foundation of East Asian thought. Nonetheless, it is still a 2000 year old system that becomes increasingly difficult to reconcile with modern knowledge. In contemporary Eastern medicine and martial arts, the five phases are generally only used as a simplistic way to remember organ and meridian relationships, and as a theoretical context for understanding the evolution of acupoint combinations used in healing and combat. Basing acupoint choice solely on a mechanical application of five phase theory, is likely to produce disappointing results. This type of antiquated approach is actively discouraged by most contemporary experts.

Five Phases

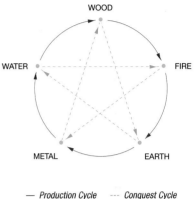

— *Production Cycle* --- *Conquest Cycle*

Phase Qualities

Wood	Growing or increasing
Fire	Maximum growth, about to decline
Metal	Declining
Water	Maximum decline, about to grow
Earth	Balanced or Neutral

Correspondences Associated with the Five Phases

	Wood	Fire	Earth	Metal	Water
Direction	East	South	Center	West	North
Season	Spring	Summer	Long Summer	Autumn	Winter
Climate	Wind	Summer Heat	Dampness	Dryness	Cold
Process	Birth	Growth	Transformation	Harvest	Storage
Color	Green	Red	Yellow	White	Black
Taste	Sour	Bitter	Sweet	Pungent	Salty
Smell	Goatish	Burning	Fragrant	Rank	Rotten
Yin Organ	Liver	Heart	Spleen	Lungs	Kidneys
Yang Organ	Gallbladder	Small Intestine	Stomach	Large Intestine	Bladder
Opening	Eyes	Tongue	Mouth	Nose	Ears
Tissue	Sinews	Blood Vessels	Flesh	Skin/Hair	Bones
Emotion	Anger	Happiness	Pensiveness	Sadness	Fear
Human Sound	Shout	Laughter	Song	Weeping	Groan

Fundamental Substances

In traditional Chinese philosophy and medicine, five fundamental properties found within the human body influence our physical, mental and emotional processes. Commonly referred to as *Fundamental Substances*, they should be thought of as concepts pertaining to bodily functions, rather than actual physical realities. Most discussion of *Fluids and Blood* within this section refers to the Eastern concept of these substances as defined below (terms are capitalized to distinguish them from their Western counterparts). This is also true of *Organs,* which will be outlined next. The five Fundamental Substances are:

- Qi (also written as Chi or Ki)
- Blood (Xue)
- Fluids (Jin Ye)
- Spirit (Shen)
- Essence (Jing)

Qi

The primal forces of yin and yang are often collectively referred to as *Qi* or *Chi* in Chinese, or *Ki* in Korean and Japanese. The word itself is essentially untranslatable, although it is often described as the "vital energy" or "life force" that permeates the universe, flowing through and animating all things. It is the basis of Eastern medicine and many healing arts. The concept of Qi is totally alien to traditional Western science, although similar concepts have been the foundation of Western occultism and native American spiritual traditions for centuries. The medical traditions of India also purport a similar energetic concept, which they call *Prana.*

Within the human body, Qi is said to have six major functions: protect the body from disease; support and sustain all movement; support body transformations; retain Fundamental Substances, organs and fluids; and maintain normal body heat. In Eastern medicine, Qi is analyzed to help determine the nature of an illness and the method of treatment. Over the last several millennia, Eastern medicine has defined various forms of Qi within the body, based on function:

Source Qi, which exists at birth, is the fundamental energy of the body. It is formed from the *Essence of the Kidneys,* the nutrients absorbed from food, and energy absorbed by the lungs from the air. It flows throughout the body and is the basis for all movement and action. In Eastern medicine its condition can be evaluated and treated using specific procedures, empirically determined through clinical observation over two thousand years. Source Qi manifests itself in different forms including Organ Qi, Channel Qi, Nourishing Qi, Protective Qi and Ancestral Qi.

Organ Qi is associated with the functions and activities of the Organs.

Channel Qi is associated with transporting and moving functions of the meridians.

Nourishing Qi (also called Blood Qi) moves with the blood, where its main purposes are creating and transforming blood, and assisting blood nourishment of body tissues.

Protective Qi circulates between the skin and flesh, where it protects the body from harmful external influences (diseases); regulates body temperature by opening and closing pores; and moistens the skin, muscles and hair. Generally, it travels throughout the superficial body during the day, while at night it is stored and circulated deep within internal organs.

Ancestral Qi is the force which transports Nourishing and Protective Qi throughout the body. It collects in the chest, where it travels upward to the throat and downward into the abdomen. The CO-17 acupoint marks its center (a vital target in most martial arts). Ancestral Qi regulates the heart beat and is involved in speaking and breathing functions. Strengthening the body by affecting Ancestral Qi, is a frequent objective of meditation.

Blood

Blood is defined as a force as well as a substance, and is linked to sense organ sensitivity. Blood is said to be created in the *middle warmer of Triple Warmer Organ,* using

Qi derived from air in the lungs, and digested food in the spleen. From there it circulates throughout the body, where its major role is nourishment of body tissues.

Fluids

Fluids are defined as sweat, urine, saliva, tears and secretions. Thick fluids are yin, and are said to moisten and nourish inner organs and the brain, and assist bone and joint movement. Thin fluids are yang, and are said to moisten muscles, skin and flesh, as well as skin at sensory and excretory openings.

Spirit (Shen)

Most cultures and religions embrace the idea that every human is animated by a divine force—often called spirit, soul or god within. In East Asian thought, this concept is called *shen* or *shin,* which roughly means *spirit.* It is believed that shen is manifest in every human in a unique and individualistic way, and is the essence which defines our inner spirit or true nature. Shen is believed to dwell in the heart where it defines our emotional and physical natures, ruling all activities of Qi in both the mind and body. It can be seen at work modulating our physical energy and emotional harmony, and guides both the intellect and the will. Shen is that part of an individual that defines his or her "essential nature" in relation to other humans. It is yang in quality.

Essence (Jing)

Spirit (a yin quality) has been defined as the force behind consciousness and thought. *Essence* (a yang quality) is defined as the force within the body that is the basis for all growth, development and sexuality. *Congenital essence* is a portion of the body's *essence* which is inherited, and determines our individual growth patterns after birth. Congenital essence can never be replaced if lost, but can be supplemented by *acquired essence,* derived from food.

In Chinese medicine, Qi, Spirit and Essence are collectively referred to as the *Three Treasures.* Harmony between these elements is considered vital to one's health and life.

Eastern Concept of the Organs

It is important to understand that the Eastern conception of *the Organs* (called viscera), radically differs from that of Western medicine, its most noticeable characteristic being that it does not adhere to actual anatomical reality. The Organ names are similar to Western terms, but do not refer to specific organ tissue. Rather, they are abstract concepts defining closely related body functions. These defined functions are based on observation of patients over a period of centuries—not on surgical research, as in the West. One of these Organ concepts, the *Triple Warmer* (also called Triple Burner), has no anatomical correlation whatsoever. This important distinction made between organs as *anatomical structures* and organs as *groupings of bodily functions,* is often misunderstood by Westerners. Understanding this difference is vitally important since Organ relationships are the fundamental concept underlying the meridian system. Efforts to relate meridian or Organ systems based on Western physiological relationships, will lead to confusion and hinder practical applications in both medicine and combat. For example, blood pressure is affected by needling points on the Large Intestine meridian; not the Heart meridian, which physiology seems to indicate.

In Eastern medicine, there are five Yin Organs (in meridian theory a sixth, the Pericardium, is added), six Yang Organs and six Curious Organs. The Yin and Yang Organ systems are the most important in defining body functions. Yin Organ systems are said to produce, transform, regulate and store Fundamental Substances. Yang Organ systems are said to receive, break down, and absorb food transformed into Fundamental Substances, and excrete unused portions. The six Curious Organs are the Brain, Marrow (bone marrow, spinal cord), Bone, Blood Vessels, Uterus and Gallbladder (the Gallbladder is also a Yang Organ). In classic literature there is little discussion regarding the function of Curious Organs. In medical practice, they play almost no importance, since their physiological functions are part of the 12 Organ systems that encompass almost all bodily functions.

EASTERN ORGAN SYSTEMS

The illustration at right is an ancient drawing depicting Organ anatomy (c. 200 BC). Ancient Eastern healers did not concern themselves with the actual physical structure of the human body. Rather, they were more concerned with its manifestations, functions and internal relationships—all of which govern whether the body exists in a balanced or unbalanced state.

In most Eastern medical systems, Organs are defined by their bodily functions, and their relationships with Fundamental Substances, other Organs, and other body systems. The harmonious interaction of these elements leads to health and wellness.

Eastern medicine recognizes the Organ systems listed at right.

Note: In this book, Eastern Organ names are capitalized to distinguish them from Western counterparts possessing the same name. For example, *Heart* is different than *heart.*

6 Yin Organs (viscus)
Lung
Spleen
Heart
Kidney
Pericardium
Liver

6 Yang Organs (bowel)
Large Intestine
Stomach
Small Intestine
Bladder
Triple Warmer
Gallbladder

6 Curious Organs
Brain
Marrow
Bone
Blood Vessels
Uterus
Gallbladder

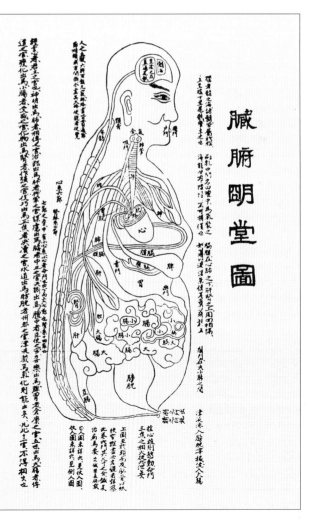

臟腑朗堂圖

THE MERIDIAN SYSTEM

Meridians (also called channels) are pathways that transport Qi, Blood and Fluids throughout the body, integrating all the body's parts into a unified whole. The system consists of 12 Regular meridians, 8 Extraordinary meridians, a network of Connecting Vessels, 12 Divergent Channels, 12 Muscle Channels and 12 Cutaneous Regions. Basically the system operates thus: 12 Regular meridians connect internally with Organs and externally with limbs and joints. Qi and Blood flow through Regular meridians and their branches (Divergent Channels and Connecting Vessels), to all parts of the body including Muscle Channels and Cutaneous Regions. When Qi is abundant, it overflows into Extraordinary meridians, where it is stored and released into Regular meridians when Qi is low.

The 12 Regular Meridians

Regular meridians are bilateral, existing on both sides of the body. Each meridian consists of an *interior pathway* lying deep within the body and connecting to an Organ (after which it is named); an *exterior pathway* running along the body's surface, delineated by acupoints; and one or more *Divergent Channels* that enter deep into body cavities.

Regular meridians are classified according to yin and yang, and the limb along which they run. Yin meridians run along the inner surface of a limb, and across the chest and abdomen. Yang meridians run along the outer surface of a limb and over the back and buttocks. Yin meridians link to upper Organs (viscus); yang meridians to lower digestive Organs (bowel).

Qi-Flow

On each Regular meridian, the Qi flows in specific directions according to specific laws. All 12 meridians are sequentially linked by *Connecting Vessels* and *Divergent Channels*. The Qi flows through the body in a 24-hour cycle (called *diurnal cycle*) that begins in the Lung meridian, and continues in a prescribed order through all Regular meridians, ending at the last point on the Liver meridian, where the cycle begins again. Qi and Blood are most concentrated in each meridian during the two hour period listed opposite. Flow timing and direction is used in both healing and combat to increase the effectiveness of techniques. For example, massaging a meridian in the direction of Qi-flow is more beneficial than the the opposite motion; and striking an acupoint which is in an "active phase" will increase the effect of the blow. This is covered later, in the chapter on *Martial Applications*.

The 8 Extraordinary Meridians

These meridians (also called vessels) function very differently than the 12 Regular meridians. They don't have a continuous, interconnected circulation of Qi-flow, nor are they associated with specific Organs. Except for the Governing and Conception meridians, they do not possess their own acupoints, but share points found on Regular meridians. Qi flows through these meridians along deep interior and superficial exterior pathways, in varying directions, as it moves between areas of Qi deficiency and Qi excess, balancing Regular meridians. These eight meridians were historically referred to as the *Strange Flows*, and are believed to be the vital meridians through which all of the body's energy-flows are interrelated. They are usually grouped into four pairs, as shown in the chart at right. These eight meridians are also the foundation of many Taoist internal practices and ancient acupuncture and massage systems. They are very affected by hand pressure or meditation, and are directly related to the Brain, Womb, Liver and Kidney (location of Source Qi).

Connecting Vessels

Connecting Vessels are branches originating from larger meridians. There are two basic subsystems. The first consists of *15 Large Connecting Vessels,* one each branching from the 12 Regular meridians, the Governing meridian, the Conception meridian, and the Great Connecting Vessel of the Spleen. Their primary function is to link the Regular meridians to their complimentary (yin-yang) meridian. They branch from Regular meridians at specific acupoints on the limbs and traverse near the body's surface. The second subsystem consists of small connecting vessels that help distribute Qi and blood throughout the body. They are called: *Minute Connecting Vessels* (branches of the 15 Large Connecting Vessels); *Superficial Connecting Vessels* (serving the body's surface, called "12 Cutaneous Regions"); and *Blood Connecting Vessels* (small and visible).

12 Regular Meridians: Names and Classification

Arm–Yin Meridians	Arm–Yang Meridians
Arm Greater Yin—Lung Meridian	Arm Yang Brightness—Large Intestine Meridian
Arm Absolute Yin—Pericardium Meridian	Arm Lesser Yang—Triple Warmer Meridian
Arm Lesser Yin—Heart Meridian	Arm Greater Yang—Small Intestine Meridian

Leg–Yin Meridians	Leg–Yang Meridians
Leg Greater Yin—Spleen Meridian	Leg Yang Brightness—Stomach Meridian
Leg Absolute Yin—Liver Meridian	Leg Lesser Yang—Gallbladder Meridian
Leg Lesser Yin—Kidney Meridian	Leg Greater Yang—Bladder Meridian

Regular meridians are named by combining their limb location, traditional yin/yang polarity and associated Organ. These long, traditional meridian names are still used in many medical texts, but are commonly shortened in the interest of brevity. For example, "Arm Greater Yin Lung Meridian" is commonly shortened to "Lung Meridian." The full name for each meridian is given above; the portion after the dash (—) indicates its abbreviated form.

12 Regular Meridians

	Symbol	Type	Phase	Acupoints	Flow Direction	Flow Timing	Connects with	Communicates with
Lung	LU	Yin	Metal	11 (x2)	Chest to Hand	3 am – 5 am	Large Intestine	Spleen
Large Intestine	LI	Yang	Metal	20 (x2)	Hand to Head	5 am – 7 am	Lung	Stomach
Stomach	ST	Yang	Earth	45 (x2)	Head to Foot	7 am – 9 am	Spleen	Large Intestine
Spleen	SP	Yin	Earth	21 (x2)	Foot to Chest	9 am – 11 am	Stomach	Lung
Heart	HT	Yin	Fire	9 (x2)	Chest to Hand	11 am – 1 pm	Small Intestine	Kidney
Small Intestine	SI	Yang	Fire	19 (x2)	Hand to Head	1 pm – 3 pm	Heart	Bladder
Bladder	BL	Yang	Water	67 (x2)	Head to Foot	3 pm – 5 pm	Kidney	Small Intestine
Kidney	KI	Yin	Water	27 (x2)	Foot to Chest	5 pm – 7 pm	Bladder	Heart
Pericardium	PC	Yin	Fire	9 (x2)	Chest to Hand	7 pm – 9 pm	Triple Warmer	Liver
Triple Warmer	TW	Yang	Fire	23 (x2)	Hand to Head	9 pm – 11 pm	Pericardium	Gallbladder
Gallbladder	GB	Yang	Wood	44 (x2)	Head to Foot	11 pm – 1 am	Liver	Triple Warmer
Liver	LV	Yin	Wood	14 (x2)	Foot to Chest	1 am – 3 am	Gallbladder	Pericardium

Note: Regular meridian names are displayed in yin-yang pairs, in the order of Qi-flow. Bilateral acupoints exist on each side of the body (x2); midline acupoints occur just once.

8 Extraordinary Meridians

	Symbol	Type	Acupoints	Flow Timing	Connects with
Conception	CO	Yin	24 midline	Anytime	6 Regular Yin Meridians
Governing	GV	Yang	28 midline	Anytime	6 Regular Yang Meridians
Penetrating		Yin	12 bilateral, 2 midline	Anytime	KI, CO, ST, (shared acupoints)
Girdling		Yang	3 bilateral	Anytime	GB, (shared acupoints)
Yin Linking		Yin	6 bilateral, 2 midline	Anytime	KI, SP, LV, CO, (shared acupoints)
Yang Linking		Yang	13 bilateral, 2 midline	Anytime	GV, GB, TW, SI, BL, (shared acupoints)
Yin Heel		Yin	3 bilateral	Anytime	BL, KI, (shared acupoints)
Yang Heel		Yang	12 bilateral, 1 midline	Anytime	GV, GB, BL, ST, LI, SI, (shared acupoints)

12 Divergent Channels

Divergent Channels are branches that diverge from each of the 12 Regular meridians and traverse the interior of the body. Their primary functions are to strengthen the yin/yang relationships between the Regular meridians (e.g., Lung-Large Intestine), distribute Qi to the face and head, and integrate otherwise unconnected parts of the body into the overall meridian system. Their importance is primarily theoretical in that their paths are used to explain the functions and connections between various acupoints, Organs and other parts of the body, not normally served by the interior/exterior paths of Regular and Extraordinary meridians. Although Divergent Channels are branches of the 12 Regular meridians, they are often considered a separate system, since they possess unique qualities and distribute Qi over a wide area.

12 Muscle Channels

Muscle Channels are groups of muscles, tendons and ligaments that follow the paths of the 12 Regular meridians after which they are named. Generally, they begin at the extremities of the limbs and ascend to the head or trunk. Muscle Channels do not possess acupoints, transport Blood or Qi, or connect to Organs. Their functions are similar to functions attributed in Western medicine to musculature. They depend upon Qi and Blood supplied by other meridians to properly function. The Muscle Channels connect and converge at various points of the body. Each Muscle Channel connects to at least one other Muscle Channel. Four sets of Muscle Channels (grouped by yin/yang, hand/foot) unite at four places: the cheek, the genital area, the corner of the forehead, and the thoracic-abdominal area.

12 Cutaneous Regions

The surface of the body (skin) is divided into "12 Cutaneous Regions" that link to and are an extension of each of the 12 Regular meridians. These surface regions are supplied by *Superficial Connecting Vessels.* In Eastern medicine, diseases are believed to enter and exit the body through Cutaneous Regions. If a disease is allowed to progress, it continues to make its way via connecting vessels and meridians, eventually reaching deep organs and tissue. If diseases are detected and treated early on, or if the body's immune systems (e.g., Protective Qi) repel the pathogens, they are driven outward to Cutaneous Regions, where they leave the body. In Eastern medicine, Cutaneous Regions are often analyzed for color, skin sensation or abnormal formations, to determine the nature and specific locations of disease.

Component Parts of a Regular Meridian

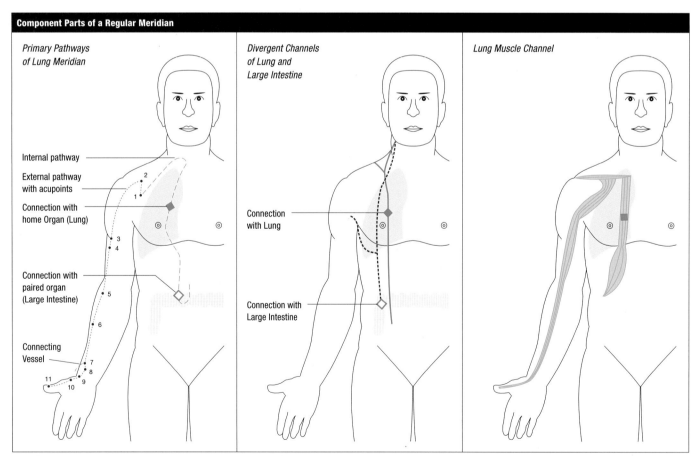

Primary Pathways of Lung Meridian

Internal pathway
External pathway with acupoints
Connection with home Organ (Lung)
Connection with paired organ (Large Intestine)
Connecting Vessel

Divergent Channels of Lung and Large Intestine

Connection with Lung
Connection with Large Intestine

Lung Muscle Channel

Drawings show the Lung system's interior and exterior pathways, Connecting Vessel, Divergent Channel, and Muscle Channel. Other Regular meridians possess similar elements.

Meridian System Summary

Meridians

12 Regular Meridians	Primary meridians circulating Qi and blood throughout the body; connect internally with Organs, externally with limbs and joints.
8 Extraordinary Meridians	Act as reservoirs balancing the meridian system; connected to Regular meridians; closely related to Brain, Womb, Liver, and Kidney.
12 Divergent Channels	Branch from and return to Regular meridians in the body's interior; distribute Qi to the head; connect yin/yang meridian pairs.

Connecting Vessels

15 Large Connecting Vessels	Branch from 14 Major meridians at acupoints on the extremities; distribute Qi and Blood; connect yin/yang meridian pairs.
Minute Connecting Vessels	Small branches of the 15 Large Connecting Vessels; help distribute Qi and Blood throughout the body.
Superficial Connecting Vessels	Branches serving the body's surface, which is organized into 12 Cutaneous Regions (related to 12 Regular meridians).
Blood Connecting Vessels	Small visible vessels near the body's surface.

Related Regions

12 Muscle Channels	Groupings of muscles, tendons and ligaments; follow paths of 12 Regular meridians; depend on Qi and Blood from other meridians.
12 Cutaneous Regions	Division of the body's surface into 12 regions; served by Superficial Connecting Vessels; related to 12 Regular meridians.
Organs	Abstract concepts defining closely related body functions, not actual anatomical structures or organs.
6 Yin Organs (viscus)	Organ systems which produce, transform, regulate and store Fundamental Substances (Qi, Blood, Fluids, Spirit and Essence).
6 Yang Organs (bowel)	Organ systems which receive, break down, and absorb food transformed into Fundamental Substances, and excrete unused portions.
6 Curious Organs	Brain, Marrow, Bones, Uterus, Blood Vessels and Gallbladder (also a yang Organ); of little importance in theory or practice.

Acupoints

Meridian Acupoints	361 acupoints located on the external paths of the 12 Regular meridians, Conception meridian and Governing meridian.
Extra Acupoints	394 acupoints located on the body's surface; majority do not lie on meridians, some do; called Miscellaneous and New Acupoints.
Bilateral Acupoints	Refers to acupoints found symmetrically on both sides of the body.
Midline Acupoints	Refers to acupoints occurring once on the body's median axis (a vertical line dividing the body into left and right halves).

12 REGULAR MERIDIANS

For most martial artists and healing practitioners, the most important portion of the 12 Regular meridians are their external pathways and acupoints. To facilitate a clearer understanding, each Regular meridian is shown individually in what is commonly called "simplified form," and numbered (1–12) according to its Qi-flow order. The internal pathways, branches, Connecting Vessels, Divergent Channels, and Muscle Channels that are also a part of each meridian are not shown, since they would add unnecessary complexity to the drawings. A complete listing of meridians and acupoints, with large detailed drawings, is found toward the end of this chapter. This reference material also includes meridian summaries, and comprehensive acupoint tables listing Chinese, Korean and Japanese names; precise anatomical locations; and corresponding nerves and blood vessels.

1 Lung
2 Large Intestine
3 Stomach
4 Spleen
5 Heart
6 Small Intestine
7 Bladder
8 Kidney
9 Pericardium
10 Triple Warmer
11 Gallbladder
12 Liver

■ Yin Meridians
■ Yang Meridians

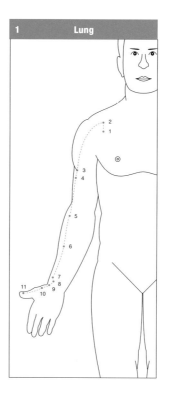

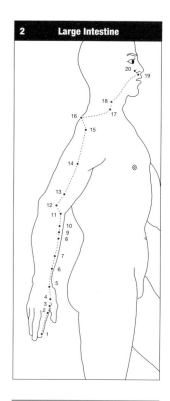

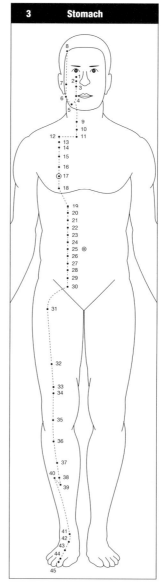

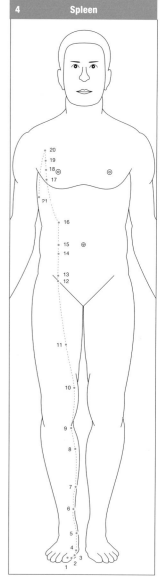

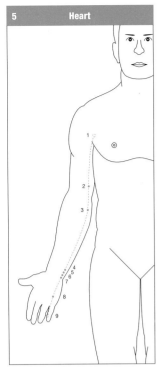

5   Heart

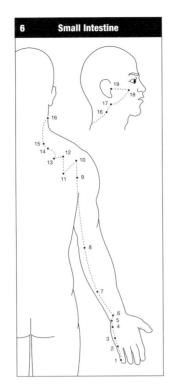

6   Small Intestine

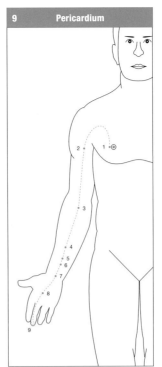

9   Pericardium

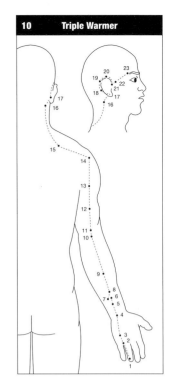

10   Triple Warmer

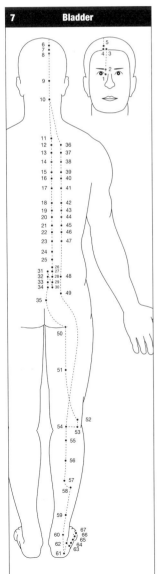

7   Bladder

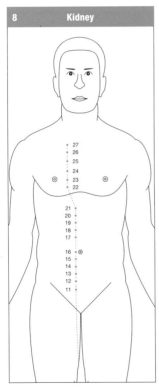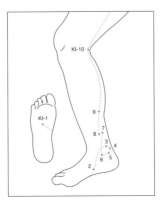

8   Kidney

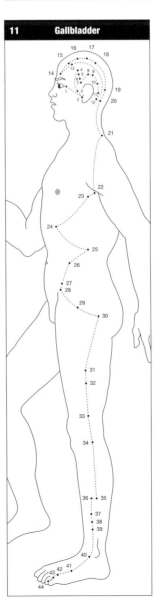

11   Gallbladder

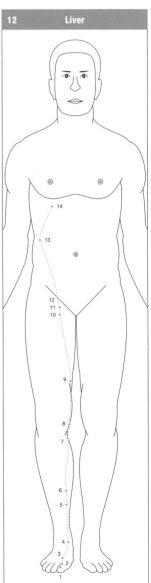

12   Liver

8 EXTRAORDINARY MERIDIANS

The drawings at right show the external pathways and acupoints of the eight Extraordinary meridians. Two of these meridians, the Conception and Governing, possess their own unique acupoints. The remaining six meridians share points found on other meridians (see list at right). Some of these shared acupoints are also shared between two or more Extraordinary meridians. A complete listing of meridians and acupoints, with large detailed drawings, is found toward the end of this chapter.

The eight Extraordinary meridians are normally grouped in pairs, which possess complimentary functions and paths.

Conception and Governing Meridians

This pair of meridians was classically called the *Great Central Channel,* and was considered the most fundamental of all Qi-flows; vital to the well-being of body and spirit. The Great Central Channel consists of the Conception meridian running down the front median line and the Governing meridian, running up the back median line. Qi flows through these meridians as it moves between areas of Qi deficiency and Qi excess, balancing the entire meridian system.

The Conception meridian, called the *Sea of Yin Meridians* or *Great Mother Flow,* regulates the six Regular yin meridians. The Governing meridian, called *Sea of Yang Meridians* or *Great Father Flow,* regulates the six Regular yang meridians. The left and right side of each Regular meridian connect at one or more points along these vessels, forming a continuous flow. All six yang meridians converge at the GV-14 acupoint.

Penetrating Meridian

The Penetrating and Girdling meridians are the most dissimilar of the Extraordinary meridian pairs, each possessing different functions and paths. The Penetrating meridian, classically called the *Sea of the Twelve Meridians*, has a regulating effect on all 12 Regular meridians. It is said to store the *true body Qi* and helps regulate development of *Pre-Natal Qi* and *Post-Natal Qi.* Classic texts state this meridian "restrains and regulates sinews [muscles and tendons] and meridians of the whole body." It is also called the *Sea of Blood* since it regulates menstruation.

In many Taoist internal practices, the Governing, Conception and Penetrating meridians are considered the three great psychic meridians, which transmit cosmic energy throughout the body—primarily through controlled breathing. Releasing and directing Qi through these three meridians generally has a calming, centering effect.

Girdling Meridian

The Girdling meridian, which resembles a belt or girdle encircling the hips, is the only meridian in which Qi flows horizontally throughout its entire pathway. Its basic function is to join all the meridians running up and down the trunk, balancing the upward and downward flow of Qi in the body. It intersects with three points on the Gallbladder meridian. Since these points are bilateral, occurring identically on left and right sides of the body, there are a total of six points on the Girdling meridian.

Yin and Yang Linking Meridians

This pair of meridians was classically called the *Great Regulator Channel,* and was considered to be "the binding network of all the vessels." The *Yin Linking meridian* connects the flows of the six Regular yin meridians (Lung, Spleen, Heart, Kidney, Pericardium, Liver), reinforcing and balancing the yin Qi-flows. It is said to control the nourishing energy of the body, and regulates the blood and interior regions. The *Yang Linking meridian* connects the flows of the six Regular yang meridians (Large Intestine, Stomach, Small Intestine, Bladder, Triple Warmer, Gallbladder), reinforcing and balancing the yang Qi-flows. It is said to control the defensive energy of the body, and regulates the exterior regions and resistance to external pathogens (the outside agents that cause diseases).

Yin and Yang Heel Meridians

This pair of meridians was classically called the *Bridge Channel,* since they act as a bridge linking yin and yang energies. They primarily control physiologic functions involving the ascent of Fluids and the descent of Qi, the opening and closing of the eyes, and general muscular activity. Qi excess in one Heel meridian usually corresponds to a Qi deficiency in the other meridian, resulting in an excess of either yin or yang energy. Disruption or blockage of Qi-flow in the Yin Heel meridian often results in fatigue or drowsiness. Qi blockages in the Yang Heel meridian often results in hypertension and insomnia.

SHARED ACUPOINTS

The six Extraordinary meridians listed below, share acupoints found on other meridians. Acupoints shared by two Extraordinary meridians are marked with an asterisk (*). These six meridians are mostly bilaterally symmetrical, occurring on both sides of thebody.

Penetrating Meridian

KI-21	KI-15
KI-20	KI-14
KI-19	KI-13
KI-18	KI-12
KI-17	KI-11
KI-16	ST-30
CO-7*	CO-1*

Girdling Meridian

GB-26
GB-27
GB-28

Yin Linking Meridian

CO-23*	SP-15
CO-22*	SP-13
LV-14	SP-12
SP-16	KI-9

Yang Linking Meridian

GV-15*	GB-14
GV-16*	GB-13
GB-20*	GB-21
GB-19	TW-15
GB-18	SI-10*
GB-17	GB-35
GB-16	BL-63
GB-15	

Yin Heel Meridian

BL-1*
KI-8
KI-6

Yang Heel Meridian

GV-16*	LI-16
GB-20*	SI-10*
BL-1*	GB-29
ST-1	BL-59
ST-3	BL-61
ST-4	BL-62
LI-15	

◉ Intersection Point with other Extraordinary meridians (see drawings)

■ Yin Meridians
■ Yang Meridians

Conception

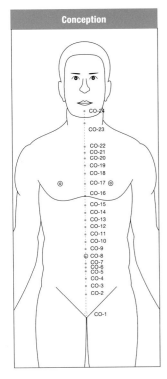

CO-24
CO-23
CO-22
CO-21
CO-20
CO-19
CO-18
CO-17
CO-16
CO-15
CO-14
CO-13
CO-12
CO-11
CO-10
CO-9
CO-8
CO-7
CO-6
CO-5
CO-4
CO-3
CO-2
CO-1

Governing

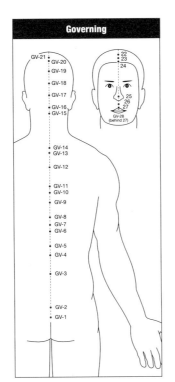

GV-21
GV-20
GV-19
GV-18
GV-17
GV-16
GV-15
GV-14
GV-13
GV-12
GV-11
GV-10
GV-9
GV-8
GV-7
GV-6
GV-5
GV-4
GV-3
GV-2
GV-1

22
23
24
25
26
27
GV-28
(behind 27)

Penetrating

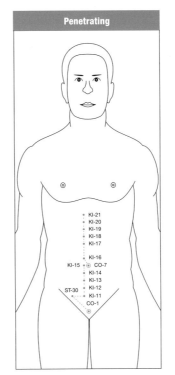

KI-21
KI-20
KI-19
KI-18
KI-17
KI-16
KI-15   CO-7
KI-14
KI-13
KI-12
ST-30   KI-11
CO-1

Girdling

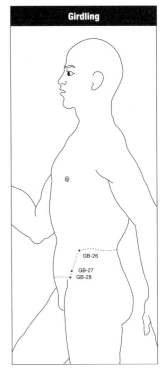

GB-26
GB-27
GB-28

Yin Linking

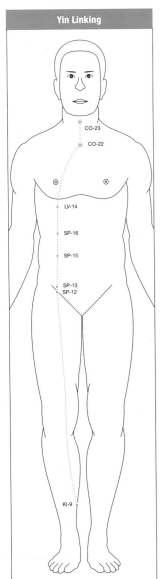

CO-23
CO-22
LV-14
SP-16
SP-15
SP-13
SP-12
KI-9

Yang Linking

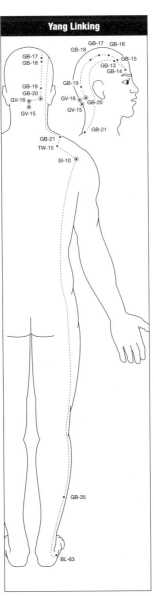

GB-17   GB-16
GB-18
GB-17   GB-15
GB-18   GB-13
GB-14
GB-19   GB-19
GB-20
GV-16   GV-16   GB-20
GV-15   GV-15
GB-21
GB-21
TW-15
SI-10
GB-35
BL-63

Yin Heel

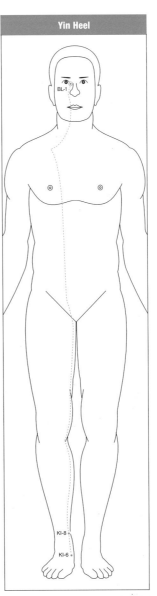

BL-1
KI-8
KI-6

Yang Heel

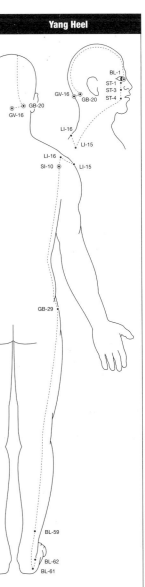

BL-1
ST-1
ST-3
ST-4
GV-16   GB-20
GB-20
GV-16
LI-16
LI-15
LI-16
SI-10   LI-15
GB-29
BL-59
BL-62
BL-61

14 MAJOR MERIDIANS

The following drawings show the external pathways and acupoints of the 12 Regular meridians and two of the eight Extraordinary meridians—the Conception and Governing meridians. Collectively they are referred to as the *14 Major meridians,* since they are the most important components of the meridian system. Common *Extra Acupoints* not directly linked to meridians are also shown. This is the standard method for visualizing the meridian system and is often reproduced in wall-size charts. The internal pathways, branches, Connecting Vessels, Divergent Channels and Muscle Channels that are also a part of each meridian are not shown, since they add too much complexity and are primarily used in medicine. Comprehensive acupuncture texts will provide additional information (see list in *Appendix*).

Drawing Notes

All 12 Regular meridians are bilateral, occurring on the left and right sides of the body. Conception and Governing meridians occur once on the body's midline. On the front and rear views, half of the drawing shows meridians only, with arrows indicating Qi-flow direction. The opposite half shows the same meridians with acupoints, identified using the standard letter/number symbol. Different systems may alter meridian placement or number points differently, particularly on the Bladder meridian, although a point's Chinese name and functions remain the same. The 14 Major meridians are found on the following views (views are listed in order of clarity):

BL	Bladder	rear, front, side
CO	Conception	front
GB	Gallbladder	side, front rear
GV	Governing	rear, front, side
HT	Heart	front, side
KI	Kidney	front, side
LI	Large Intestine	side, rear
LV	Liver	front, side
LU	Lung	front
PC	Pericardium	front
SI	Small Intestine	rear, side
SP	Spleen	front, side
ST	Stomach	front, side
TW	Triple Warmer	rear, side

- ● Meridian Acupoint
- ○ Extra Acupoint
- ◇ Acupoint Beyond
- ---- Meridian Path
- — Body Surfaces
- ◄ Qi-Flow Direction
- ■ Yin Meridians
- ■ Yang Meridians

BL	Bladder
CO	Conception
GB	Gallbladder
GV	Governing
HT	Heart
KI	Kidney
LI	Large Intestine
LV	Liver
LU	Lung
PC	Pericardium
SI	Small Intestine
SP	Spleen
ST	Stomach
TW	Triple Warmer

Note:

For purposes of clarity, meridians are also shown individually on the preceding pages.

Larger detailed drawings of individual meridians are provided later in this chapter.

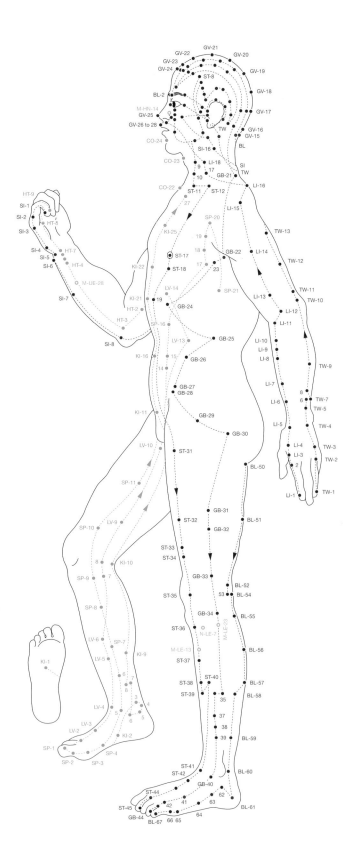

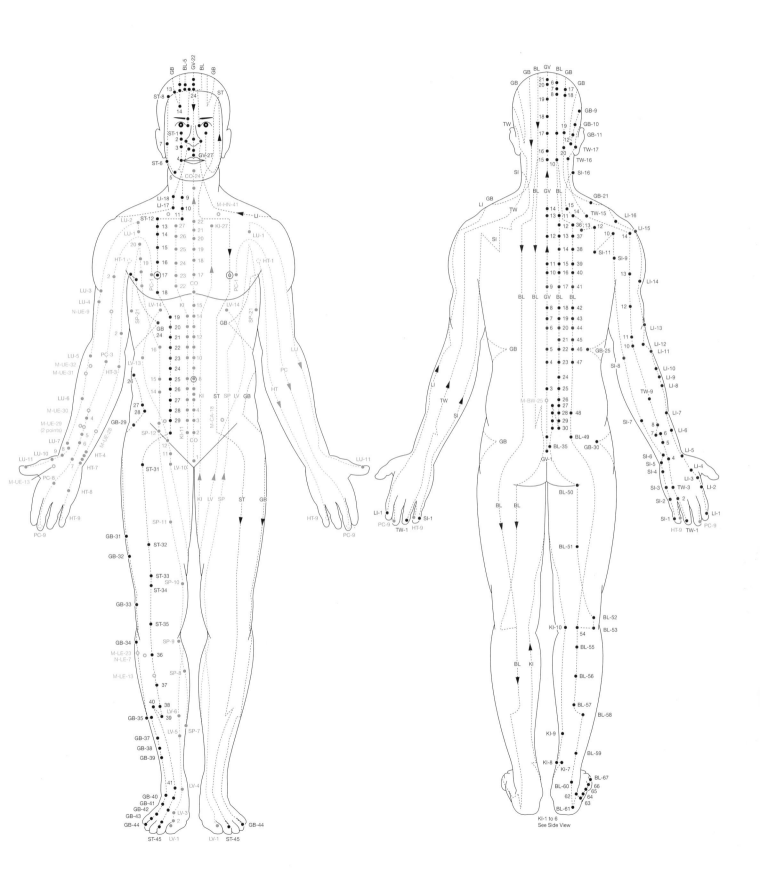

ACUPOINTS

ACUPOINTS

Eastern medicine has currently identified over 2000 acupoints on the human body, although few systems make use of this many different points. The specific points used depends on the system. Acupuncture makes use of more points than massage, since points affected by needling are far greater in number than those affected by finger pressure.

Currently, most acupuncture systems consist of 361 *Meridian acupoints* located on the external paths of the 12 Regular meridians, Conception meridian and Governing meridian; and 394 *Extra acupoints,* most of which do not lie on meridians. Some of these points do in fact lie on the 12 Regular meridians, but theoreticians unwilling to renumber or add to the existing 361 points have classified them differently. Points found symmetrically on both sides of body are called *bilateral points.* Points occurring once on the body's median axis (a vertical line dividing body into left and right halves) are called *midline points.* Extra acupoints occur either once or twice, depending on the point and its placement.

12 Regular Meridians (bilateral):	309 Points
Conception/Governing Meridians (midline):	52 Points
Extra Acupoints:	394 Points
Total:	755 Points

Acupoints were discovered gradually over a period of centuries based on a process of trial and observation. By AD 300, over 95 percent of the 361 Meridian acupoints had been identified. Since the 1950s, many new points have been found on major nerve trunks and branches, and around the eyes, ears and lower limbs, by combining traditional meridian theory with Western anatomical descriptions of body systems. New acupoints have also been located using electrical probes to measure electrical conductivity of the skin, which has led to the discovery of many "electrically excitable" motor points in nerves and muscles. Many of these new points have highly specialized medical applications such as treating paralysis, deafness, mutism and eye disorders.

Acupoint Names

Historically acupoint names evolved as a representation of natural world phenomena, related by metaphor to the geography of the body. These names, rich in meaning and imagery, were used to remember medical theories, locations, effects, and energetic relationships associated with each acupoint. This terminology is still in use today. Later, an alphanumeric system of letters and numbers evolved to shorten and simplify acupoint names into a universal system. *Meridian acupoints* are identified with letters designating the meridian, and sequential numbers designating specific points. Acupoint numbers increase in the direction of Qi-flow. In *Extra acupoints,* letters refer to anatomical position. For example, M-LE-13 is a Miscellaneous point on the Lower Extremity.

Unfortunately, the alphanumeric system is not used consistently. Different texts use different abbreviations or numbering. Later in this chapter, tables cross-reference each acupoint with its Chinese, Korean and Japanese name, and its anatomical location. This permits verification with other systems and texts.

Acupoint Functions

The nature and function of acupoints have been determined by location, the meridian to which they belong, by special groupings they are part of, and from clinical observations by medical practitioners and martial artists, for over two millennia. Medical texts will provide detailed tables outlining acupoint uses and effects. Of the 755 points outlined at left, less than 200 are commonly used by most martial artists and healing practitioners.

Stimulation of an acupoint manipulates Qi-flow in the immediate area of that point, affecting surrounding muscles, tissue, joints, or organs—or if the point is prominently located, can effect an entire region of the body. For example, points in the immediate area of the knee can be used to either heal a painful joint or damage a healthy one. The CO-12 acupoint on the Conception meridian is close to the stomach and is often used to

affect its condition. Prominently located points such as CO-17 on sternum can affect the entire chest region, including deep organs. Its importance results from the fact that it is an intersection point of four meridians (SP, SI, KI, TW), an important diagnostic point (*Alarm-Mu Point*) for the Pericardium, and one of the eight important points influencing Qi (*Meeting-Hui Point*). In healing, it is used to treat stomach and intestinal disorders. In martial arts, it is a vital target found in many systems.

Special Acupoint Groupings

Many acupoints belong to one or more special groupings, each characterized by special relationships to meridians and connecting vessels. Common groups are:

12 Source-Yuan Points

These are the points located on each of the 12 Regular meridians where the Source Qi resides and is regulated. They are closely linked to the Triple Warmer.

15 Connecting-Luo Points

These are points at which connecting vessels branch from major meridians. A single point is possessed by each of the 12 Regular meridians, and the Conception and Governing meridians. Two points are associated with the Spleen, one for each of its two Connecting Vessels: Spleen Connecting Vessel (SP-4), and the Great Connecting Vessel of Spleen (SP-21).

16 Cleft-Xi Points

These are points where Qi accumulates as it circulates through the meridians. A small cleft (indent) is felt at the point's location, and is often sensitive when Qi is in excess (swollen, red) or depletion (dull pain, indented). One point is located on each of the 12 Regular meridians and on four Extraordinary meridians (Yin and Yang Linking, Yin and Yang Heel).

8 Meeting-Hui Points

Each point affects the specific body element shown in the chart. They are often combined with other points to treat specific problems and were identified by the ancient Chinese during centuries of clinical observation.

4 Command Points

These points command specific body regions and were identified as early as the fourteenth century. In medicine, they are used to treat afflictions stemming from the area they serve.

12 Alarm-Mu Points

These are points on the chest and abdomen where meridian Qi collects, from each Regular meridian (also called collection points). They are located directly above or near their related Organ. In medicine, they primarily function as diagnostic tools, alerting the healer to an abnormal condition or pathogen. They are often used to treat disorders relating to the six bowel Organs.

12 Associated-Shu Points

These points are located on the Bladder meridian, along the portion of its path running parallel to the spine. Each Shu Point is the place where Qi passes on its way to a particular Organ. In Eastern medicine, such points are primarily used to diagnose and treat the related Organ after which they are named (e.g., Heart Shu, Lung Shu, etc.).

6 Lower Uniting-He Points

In the head, the three yang meridians beginning in the hand (LI, SI, TW) connect with the three yang meridians terminating in the foot (ST, BL, GB). There is one acupoint representing each of the six yang meridians.

Special Acupoint Groupings

	Source Point	Connecting Point	Cleft Point	Alarm Point	Associated Point	Lower Uniting	
Lung ---	LU-9	LU-7	LU-6	LU-1	BL-13		*Note:*
Large Intestine —	LI-4	LI-6	LI-7	ST-25	BL-25	ST-37	*Regular meridian*
Stomach —	ST-42	ST-40	ST-34	CO-12	BL-21	ST-36	*or Organ names are displayed in*
Spleen ---	SP-3	SP-4, SP-21	SP-8	LV-13	BL-20		*yin-yang pairs, in the order of*
Heart ---	HT-7	HT-5	HT-6	CO-14	BL-15		*Qi-flow.*
Small Intestine —	SI-4	SI-7	SI-6	CO-4	BL-27	ST-39	*Yang —*
Bladder —	BL-64	BL-58	BL-63	CO-3	BL-28	BL-54	*Yin ---*
Kidney ---	KI-3	KI-4	KI-5	GB-25	BL-23		
Pericardium ---	PC-7	PC-6	PC-4	CO-17	BL-14		
Triple Warmer —	TW-4	TW-5	TW-7	CO-5	BL-22	BL-53	
Gallbladder —	GB-40	GB-37	GB-36	GB-24	BL-19	GB-34	
Liver ---	LV-3	LV-5	LV-6	LV-14	BL-18		
Conception ---		CO-15					
Governing —		GV-1					
Yin Linking ---			KI-9				
Yang Linking —			GB-35				
Yin Heel ---			KI-8				
Yang Heel —			BL-59				

8 Meeting-Hui Points

LV-13	Yin Organs
CO-12	Yang Organs
CO-17	Qi
BL-17	Blood
GB-34	Muscles, Tendons
GB-39	Marrow
BL-11	Bones
LU-9	Blood Vessels

4 Command Points

ST-36	Abdomen
BL-54	Back (upper/lower)
LU-7	Head, back of neck
LI-4	Face, mouth

Intersection-Jiaohui Points

	Lung	Large Intestine	Stomach	Spleen	Heart	Small Intestine	Bladder	Kidney	Pericardium	Triple Warmer	Gallbladder	Liver	Conception	Governing	Penetrating	Girdling	Yin Linking	Yang Linking	Yin Heel	Yang Heel
BL-1			●			●	○												●	●
BL-11						●	○													
BL-12							○							●						
BL-31							○				●									
BL-34							○				●									
BL-36[41]						●	○													
BL-53							○			●										
BL-59,61,62							○													●
BL-63							○											●		
CO-1													○	●	●					
CO-2												●	○							
CO-3				●				●	●			●	○							
CO-4				●				●	●			●	○							
CO-7													○		●					
CO-10				●									○							
CO-12			●			●				●			○							
CO-13			●			●							○							
CO-17				●		●		●		●			○							
CO-22, 23													○2				●2			
CO-24			●										○							
GB-1						●				●	○									
GB-3		●								●	○									
GB-4		●								●	○									
GB-6		●								●	○									
GB-7							●				○									
GB-8							●				○									
GB-10							●				○									
GB-11							●				○									
GB-12							●				○									
GB-13, 14											○2							●2		
GB-15							●				○							●		
GB-16 to 19											○4							●4		
GB-20											○							●		●
GB-21										●	○							●		
GB-24				●							○									
GB-26 to 28											○3					●3				
GB-29											○									●
GB-30							●				○									
GB-35											○							●		
GV-1								●			●			○						
GV-13							●							○						
GV-14		●	●			●	●			●	●			○						
GV-15														○				●		

44

Intersection-Jiaohui Points

	Lung ---	Large Intestine —	Stomach —	Spleen —	Heart ---	Small Intestine —	Bladder —	Kidney ---	Pericardium ---	Triple Warmer —	Gallbladder —	Liver ---	Conception ---	Governing —	Penetrating ---	Girdling —	Yin Linking ---	Yang Linking —	Yin Heel ---	Yang Heel —
GV-16														○				●		●
GV-17							●							○						
GV-20							●							○						
GV-24			●				●							○						
GV-26		●	●											○						
GV-28													●	○						
KI-6, 8								○											●	
KI-9								○									●			
KI-11 to 21								○11							●11					
LI-15, 16		○2																		●2
LU-1	○			●																
LV-13											●	○								
LV-14				●								○					●			
PC-1									○		●									
SI-10						○												●		●
SI-12		●				○				●	●									
SI-17						○					●									
SI-18						○				●										
SI-19						○				●	●									
SP-6				○				●				●								
SP-12				○								●					●			
SP-13				○								●					●			
SP-15, 16				○2													●2			
ST-1		○											●							●
ST-3		○																		●
ST-4		●	○																	●
ST-5			○								●									
ST-7			○								●									
ST-8			○								●									
ST-12		●	○								●									
ST-30			○												●					
ST-37		●	○																	
ST-39			○			●														
TW-15										○								●		●
TW-17										○	●									
TW-20		●								○	●									
TW-22						●				○	●									

Intersection-Jiaohui Points: These are acupoints where two or more meridians intersect. Manipulation of these points affects all meridians to which the point is connected. There are about 100 points, although different medical sources vary as to quantity and the exact points used.

This chart can be used in two ways:
1. To determine which points influence a particular meridian, find the meridian name and read down.
2. To determine which meridians are influenced by a particular point, find the acupoint name and read across.

The meridian which the acupoint belongs to is called the *origin meridian*. Other meridians which intersect at this point are called *intersecting meridians*. In the chart, meridians are displayed in yin-yang pairs, in order of Qi-flow. Acupoints are in alphabetical order.

○　Origin Meridian
●　Intersecting Meridian
--- Yin Meridian
— Yang Meridian

Locating Acupoints

Acupoints are usually located in depressions at bones, joints and muscles. The area affecting each acupoint is usually the size of a dime, but can be as small as a pin head. Some acupoints are easy to locate by simply probing around, since they are very sensitive to pressure. Others are well hidden and require very precise targeting. The angle of insertion or attack is often critical. Feel for a slight depression or hollow at each point. This might be a perceived as a slight depression in the bone, a small space between muscle fibers, or a slight opening between tendons and muscles. When Qi-flow is obstructed, this depression may be hard to locate, but will often feel hard to the touch. When in doubt, martial artists will often drive a point toward bone, as this is usually more painful.

Location Methods

In ancient China, a system using body landmarks and a relative unit of measurement called a *cun,* assisted practitioners in locating acupoints. This system is still in use today. A cun (also called a body inch, unit, or finger unit) varies in length based on the proportion and size of the individual being measured. The length or width of different parts of the fingers are used to make rough estimates of acupoint locations, as shown below. Modern texts have attempted to provide greater clarity by using anatomical terminology when describing point locations. In truth, locating acupoints requires a sensitivity which can only be acquired through practical training and experience, making it as much an art as a science. After learning the general placement of meridians and acupoints, you might want to spend at least a few hours with an acupuncturist. Professional assistance can be enormously useful in helping to clarify precise acupoint locations.

Relation Between Acupoints, Nerves and Blood Vessels

Beginning about 1959, Chinese medical schools began conducting research to correlate acupoint locations with nerves and blood vessels. Based on anatomical dissections, they found that 323 points were supplied by nerves. Of these points, 304 were related to superficial cutaneous nerves (near the body's surface), 155 to deep nerves, and 137 maintained both superficial and deep neural links. Examination of points under a microscope revealed that all layers of skin and muscle tissue at these points possessed numerous and varied nerve branches, plexi (nerve networks), and nerve endings. Researchers also found that the meridian paths found on the limbs closely corresponded with the routes of peripheral nerves. For example, the Lung meridian path on the arm is similar to the route of the musculocutaneous nerve, the Pericardium meridian relates to the median nerve, and the Heart meridian relates to the routes of the ulnar and medial cutaneous nerves of arm.

Research comparing acupoints and blood vessels found that 24 points were located directly over arterial branches, 262 within 0.5 cm of either arterial or venous branches.

Acupoint Selection

There are many methods of selecting points to influence specific regions of the body. Most of these methods utilize reference charts found in detailed acupuncture texts. This applies to both healing and martial applications. The most common methods are:

- Selection of local, adjacent or distant points, based on region to be affected (see chart at right)

- Selection according to affected meridian (see reference charts in acupuncture texts)

- Selection according to empirical data and clinical experience of past generations (usually by using symptom based charts)

- Selection from *Special Point Groupings,* based on desired effect (see reference charts in acupuncture texts)

Combining Acupoints

Two or more acupoints are often combined to increase the effectiveness and efficiency of a particular medical or martial procedure. This is based on the following principles:

- Combine local points with distant points, known to affect the desired region.

- Combine points on the front and back of body (often Alarm-Mu points and Associated-Shu points).

- Combine points on yin-yang related meridians; often Source-Yuan points and Connecting-Luo points.

- Combine points on upper and lower body (this is based on yin/yang principles).

- Combine Cleft-Xi points and Meeting-Hui points, based on region to be affected.

- Combine both bilateral points (usually to affect the head, trunk, internal organs or both sides of the body).

Generally speaking, increasing the number of points in a procedure increases the effect on the body. In martial arts, this increases the effectiveness and intensity of an attack.

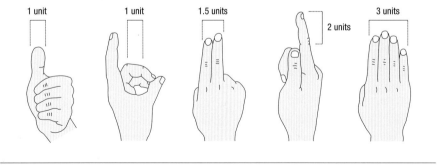

The Scientific Basis for Meridians

Currently, there is no universally proven and accepted scientific theory explaining the material basis for the meridian/acupoint system. In recent decades, extensive research and clinical practice has led in many promising directions. At this time, extensive involvement with the entire nervous system is suspected, based on extensive research correlating neural relationships between meridians and the brain, cerebral cortex, internal organs, spinal cord, motor nerves, sensory nerves, and autonomic nerves. Some researchers have also speculated that although meridians are closely related to the nervous system, they may in fact constitute a related but independent and unidentified system of conduction. Biochemical and bioelectrical activity has been measured and associated with a wide range of body tissues for decades, leading some researchers to suggest that meridians are in fact electrical pathways within the human body. As Eastern and Western medical approaches continue to evolve and merge, so will our understanding of these systems.

Summary

The preceding chapter has been an extremely brief introduction to a very vast and complex subject—the foundations of Eastern medicine. It must be understood that meridian theory and Eastern concepts of the body were developed over a period of centuries, and were the best attempt by individuals of their day to understand the workings of the human body. Some of these concepts are outdated and only used by individuals devoted to traditional practices. Others concepts have remained valid, or continue to evolve, in both *traditional* and *modern* approaches to Eastern medicine. While extensive research during preceding decades has validated many of the effects associated with meridians, there still remains a great deal of phenomena, which cannot be adequately explained within the limited framework of contemporary Western science. As our science evolves and research continues, so will our understanding of the material mechanisms at work.

Acupoint Selection Based on Region to be Affected [1]

Region Affected	Local Points	Adjacent Points	Distant Points
Eyes	BL-1, ST-1	ST-2, GV-23, M-HN-9	GB-37, LI-4, LV-3, SI-6
Ears	GB-2, SI-19, TW-17	GB-8, GB-20, SI-17	GB-41, TW-3, TW-5
Nose	LI-20, GV-25	BL-7, GV-23, M-HN-3	LI-3, LI-4, ST-44
Mouth	ST-4, ST-6, ST-7	GB-20, M-HN-9	HT-5, LI-4, ST-44, GV-15
Throat	CO-23	CO-22, SI-17	LI-4, LI-11, KI-6
Head (frontal area)	GB-14, M-HN-3	BL-5, GB-15, M-HN-9	LI-3, LI-4; ST-41, 43, 44
Head (temporal area)	GB-8, M-HN-9		GB-41, TW-3
Head (occipital area)	BL-10, GB-20		BL-65, SI-3
Vertex (top of head)	GV-20, BL-7	GB-20, M-HN-9	GB-34, LV-3
Lungs	BL-13, LU-1, CO-17, CO-22	CO-6, CO-12, GV-14	LU-5, LU-7, ST-40
Heart	BL-14, BL-15, CO-17	CO-14, GV-11	HT-7, PC-4, PC-5, PC-6
Spleen, Stomach	CO-12, BL-20, BL-21	LV-13, SP-15	PC-6, SP-4, ST-36
Liver	BL-18, LV-14	BL-20, CO-12	GB-34, LV-3
Gallbladder	BL-19, GB-24	ST-21, CO-11	GB-34+40, LV-3, M-LE-23
Large Intestine	SP-15	BL-25, ST-25	LI-11, ST-36, ST-37
Small Intestine	CO-4, CO-9, ST-28	BL-27	SI-4, ST-36, ST-39
Kidney	BL-23, BL-47[52]	ST-29, CO-4	KI-3, SP-6
Bladder	CO-3, BL-28	BL-23, ST-28	KI-3, KI-7, SP-6
Urogenital	CO-4, ST-29, M-CA-18	BL-23, BL-32	KI-3, LV-3, SP-6
Rectum	BL-35, CO-1, GV-1	BL-30, BL-34, BL-49	BL-57, GV-20, M-UE-29
Lateral Costal Region	GB-25, GB-26	LV-14, SP-21	GB-38, GB-43, TW-5
Upper Abdomen	CO-12, CO-13	CO-8, ST-19	ST-36, SP-4, PC-6
Lower Back	BL-23, GV-4	GB-25, GB-30	BL-54, BL-60, SI-3, SI-6
Shoulder	LI-15, SI-9	LI-14	LI-4, ST-38
Upper Limb	LI-4, LI-11, LI-15	M-HN-41	M-BW-35[2] (vertebra C5 to T1)
Lower Limb	GB-34, GB-39, BL-54	GB-30	M-BW-35[2] (vertebra L3 to S1)

1) This chart lists local, adjacent and distant acupoints that are often used, singularly or in combination, to treat various disease locations on the body. The same relationships can also be applied to combat.

2) M-BW-35 is a series of 48 acupoints located on both sides of the spine, at each of the 24 cervical, thoracic and lumbar vertebra, 0.5–1 unit lateral to midline, at lower end of spinous process of each vertebra.

ACUPOINT CHARTS

Front View

- ● Meridian Acupoint
- ○ Extra Acupoint
- ◌ Acupoint Beyond
- --- Meridian Path
- — Body Surfaces
- ◄ Qi-Flow Direction

- ● Major acupoint
- ○ targets are
- ◌ shown in red.

BL	Bladder
CO	Conception
GB	Gallbladder
GV	Governing
HT	Heart
KI	Kidney
LI	Large Intestine
LV	Liver
LU	Lung
PC	Pericardium
SI	Small Intestine
SP	Spleen
ST	Stomach
TW	Triple Warmer

All 12 Regular meridians are bilateral, occurring on left and right sides of the body. Conception and governing meridians occur once on body's midline.

On front and rear views, half of drawing shows meridians only, with arrows indicating Qi-flow direction. Opposite half shows same meridians with acupoints, identified using the standard letter/number symbol. Different systems may alter meridian placement or number points differently, particularly on the Bladder meridian (see list opposite).

Anatomical descriptions of point locations are listed on later pages, along with their Chinese, Korean and Japanese names.

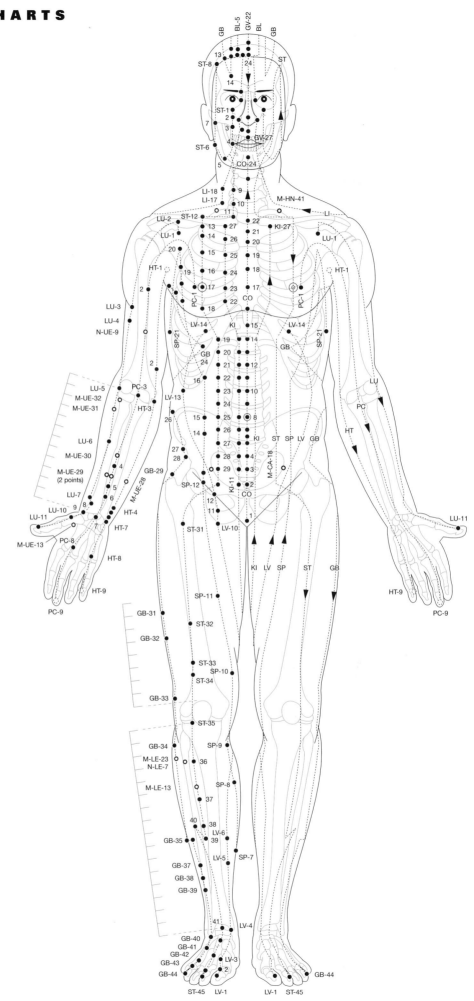

48

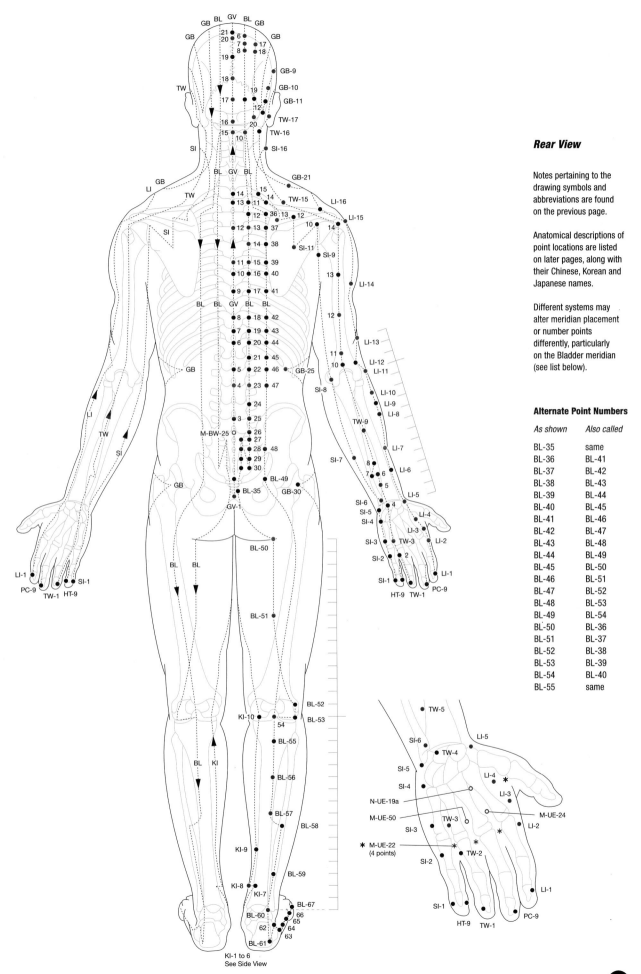

ACUPOINT CHARTS

Side View

Symbol	Meaning
●	Meridian Acupoint
○	Extra Acupoint
◇	Acupoint Beyond
----	Meridian Path
—	Body Surfaces
◄	Qi-Flow Direction

● Major acupoint
○ targets are
○ shown in red.

BL   Bladder
CO   Conception
GB   Gallbladder
GV   Governing
HT   Heart
KI   Kidney
LI   Large Intestine
LV   Liver
LU   Lung
PC   Pericardium
SI   Small Intestine
SP   Spleen
ST   Stomach
TW   Triple Warmer

All 12 Regular meridians are bilateral, occurring on left and right sides of the body. Conception and governing meridians occur once on body's midline.

Acupoints are identified using the standard letter/number symbol. Different systems may alter meridian placement or number points differently, particularly on the Bladder meridian (see list on previous page).

Anatomical descriptions of point locations are listed on later pages, along with their Chinese, Korean and Japanese names.

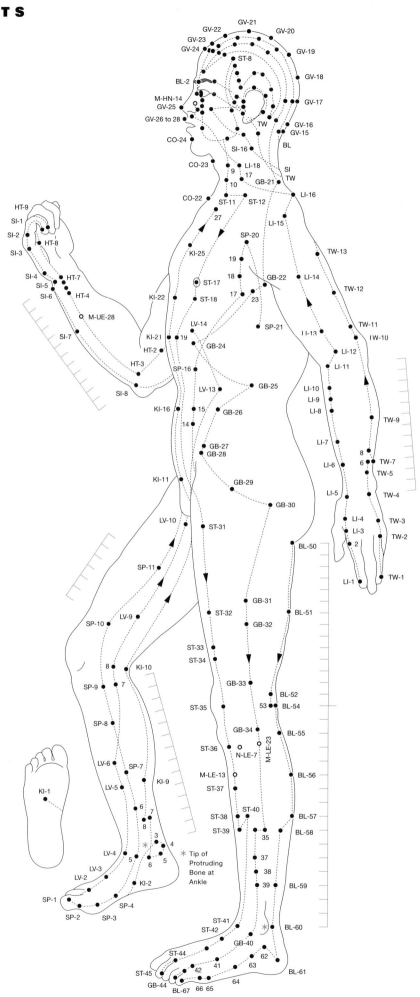

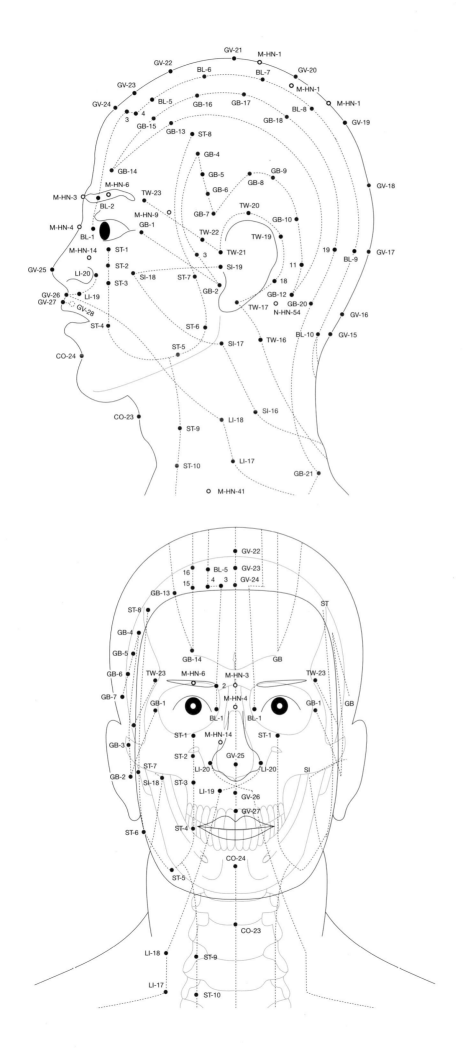

Head and Neck

These drawings identify common acupoints located on the head and neck. Some of these points were not shown on the full-body drawings, due to size limitations.

Notes pertaining to the drawing symbols and abbreviations are found on the previous page.

Anatomical descriptions of point locations are listed on later pages, along with their Chinese, Korean and Japanese names.

Contents

The following pages contain detailed drawings, tables and summaries for the twenty meridians outlined previously. The 12 Regular meridians are organized in their Qi-flow order (1–12). The 8 Extraordinary meridians are presented in complimentary pairs, and are numbered E1–E8. Extra acupoints (not generally associated with meridians) are given last.

Chinese, Korean and Japanese

The names of meridians and acupoints are given in alphanumeric code, English, Romanized Chinese (Pinyin system), Romanized Korean (Ministry of Education system), and Romanized Japanese (Hepburn system). For each entry in the following tables, Korean is on the top line, and Japanese is on the bottom line. Acupoint names written in Chinese characters are found on pages 136–139.

Key to Symbols

- ● Meridian Acupoint
- ○ Extra Acupoint
- ◌ Acupoint Beyond
- ▲ Intersection Acupoint
- ⋯⋯ External Meridian Path
- – – Internal Meridian Path
- — Body Surfaces
- ◄— Qi-Flow Direction
- ◆ Home Organ
- ◇ Paired Organ

- ● Major acupoint
- ○ targets are
- ◌ shown in red.

Proportional Scale: each space equals 1 unit (also called finger unit, body inch, or cun; see page 46)

Dashes after meridian names designate:
Yin Meridian ---
Yang Meridian —

Meridians

	English Name	Symbol	Chinese Name and English Translation	Korean (top line), Japanese (bottom line)	Points	Total Points
1	**Lung Meridian**	LU	Shou Tai Yin - Fei Jing Arm Greater Yin - Lung Channel	Su Tae Yin - Pye Gyeong Te Tai In - Hai Kei	11 bilateral	22 total
2	**Large Intestine Meridian**	LI	Shou Yang Ming - Da Chang Jing Arm Yang Brightness - Large Intestine Channel	Su Yang Myeong - Dae Jang Gyeong Te Yo Mei - Dai Cho Kei	20 bilateral	40 total
3	**Stomach Meridian**	ST	Zu Yang Ming - Wei Jing Leg Yang Brightness - Stomach Channel	Jog Yang Myeong - Wi Gyeong Ashi Yo Mei - I Kei	45 bilateral	90 total
4	**Spleen Meridian**	SP	Zu Tai Yin - Pi Jing Leg Greater Yin - Spleen Channel	Jog Tae Yin - Bi Gyeong Ashi Tai In - Hi Kei	21 bilateral	42 total
5	**Heart Meridian**	HT	Shou Shao Yin - Xin Jing Arm Lesser Yin - Heart Channel	Su So Yin - Sim Gyeong Te Sho In - Shin Kei	9 bilateral	18 total
6	**Small Intestine Meridian**	SI	Shou Tai Yang - Xiao Chang Jing Arm Greater Yang - Small Intestine Channel	Su Tae Yang - So Jang Gyeong Te Tai Yo - Sho Cho Kei	19 bilateral	38 total
7	**Bladder Meridian**	BL	Zu Tai Yang - Pang Guang Jing Leg Greater Yang - Bladder Channel	Jo Tae Yang - Bang Gwang Gyeong Ashi Tai Yo - Bo Ko Kei	67 bilateral	134 total
8	**Kidney Meridian**	KI	Zu Shao Yin - Shen Jing Leg Lesser Yin - Kidney Channel	Jog So Yin - Sin Gyeong Ashi Sho In - Jin Kei	27 bilateral	54 total
9	**Pericardium Meridian**	PC	Shou Jue Yin - Xin Bao Jing Arm Absolute Yin - Pericardium Channel	Su Gweol Yin - Sim Po Gyeong Te Ketsu In - Shin Ho Kei	9 bilateral	18 total
10	**Triple Warmer Meridian**	TW	Shou Shao Yang - San Jiao Jing Arm Lesser Yang - Triple Warmer Channel	Su So Yang - Sam Cho Gyeong Te Sho Yo - San Sho Kei	23 bilateral	46 total
11	**Gallbladder Meridian**	GB	Zu Shao Yang - Dan Jing Leg Lesser Yang - Gallbladder Channel	Jog So Yang - Dam Gyeong Ashi Sho Yo - Tan Kei	44 bilateral	88 total
12	**Liver Meridian**	LV	Zu Jue Yin - Gan Jing Leg Absolute Yin - Liver Channel	Jog Gweol Yin - Gan Gyeong Ashi Ketsu In - Kan Kei	14 bilateral	28 total
E1	**Conception Meridian**	CO	Ren Mai Conception Vessel	Im Maeg Nin Kei	24 midline	24 total
E2	**Governing Meridian**	GV	Du Mai Governing Vessel	Dog Maeg Toku Kei	28 midline	28 total
E3	**Penetrating Meridian**		Chong Mai Penetrating Vessel	Chung Maeg Sho Kei	12 bilateral 2 midline	26 total
E4	**Girdling Meridian**		Dai Mai Girdling Vessel	Dae Maeg Tai Kei	3 bilateral	6 total
E5	**Yin Linking Meridian**		Yin Wei Mai Yin Linking Vessel	Eum Yu Maeg In I Kei	6 bilateral 2 midline	14 total
E6	**Yang Linking Meridian**		Yang Wei Mai Yang Linking Vessel	Yang Yu Maeg Yo I Kei	13 bilateral 2 midline	28 total
E7	**Yin Heel Meridian**		Yin Chiao Mai Yin Heel Vessel	Eum Gyo Maeg In Kyo Kei	3 bilateral	6 total
E8	**Yang Heel Meridian**		Yang Chiao Mai Yang Heel Vessel	Yang Gyo Maeg Yo Kyo Kei	12 bilateral 1 midline	25 total

Terms Used in This Reference

Superior:	Toward the head or upper part of a structure.	Proximal:	Nearer to the attachment of an extremity, to trunk or a structure.
Inferior:	Away from head, or toward lower part of a structure.	Distal:	Farther from the attachment of an extremity, to trunk or a structure.
Anterior:	Nearer to, or at the front of body.	Superficial:	Toward or on the surface of body.
Posterior:	Nearer to, or at the back of body.	Deep:	Away from the surface of body
Medial:	Nearer to the midline of body, or a structure.	Unit:	Relative unit of measurement based on use of the fingers (cun).
Lateral:	Farther from the midline of body, or a structure.	(•)	Denotes major acupoint target

Abbreviations: (m.) muscle, (n.) nerve, (a.) artery, (v.) vein   (—) yang meridian, (---) yin meridian

Lung (LU)

Primary Paths

The Lung meridian begins internally, in the middle part of the body cavity (called the "middle warmer"), and descends to connect with the Large Intestine. Turning upward, it ascends through the diaphragm to enter its home Organ, the Lung. It continues up into the throat, turns outward and down, and emerges to the surface. The external pathway begins at the upper-outer chest (LU-1), descends the inner arm, ending at the outer corner of the thumbnail (LU-11). The Lung's Connecting Vessel branches from the primary path at LU-7, and runs to the radial tip of the forefinger to connect with the Large Intestine meridian.

Function

Lung acupoints influence the nose, throat, trachea, chest, lungs and skin, and relate to the functions of the respiratory and nervous systems.

Key Data

Type:	Yin
Phase:	Metal
Acupoints:	11 (x2)
Qi-Flow:	3 am – 5 am
Connects with:	Large Intestine
Communication:	Spleen

Special Points

Source-Yuan:	LU-9
Connecting-Luo:	LU-7
Cleft-Xi:	LU-6
Alarm-Mu:	LU-1
Associated-Shu:	BL-13
Meeting-Hui (Blood Vessels):	LU-9
Command (head, rear neck):	LU-7

Intersection-Jiaohui Points

Spleen ---	LU-1

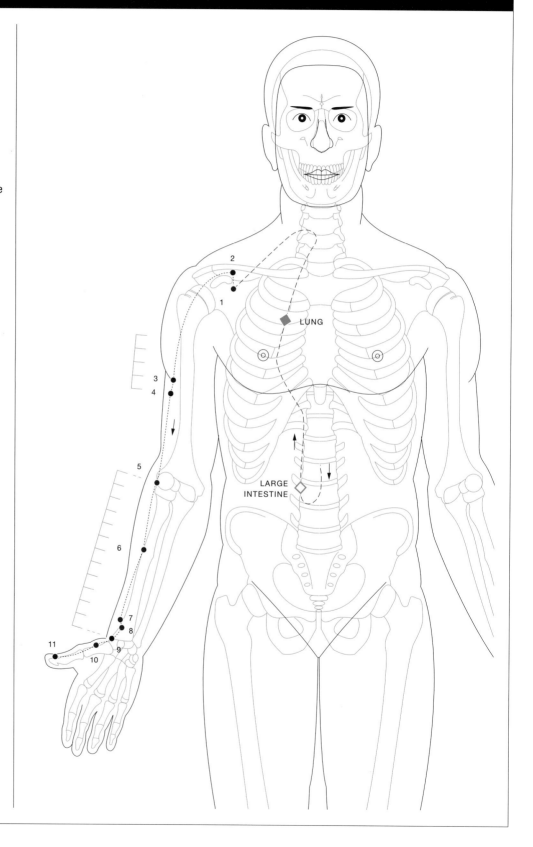

Lung (LU)

Symbol	Chinese Name	Korean Japanese	Location	Local Anatomy (Nerves and Blood Vessels)
• LU-1	Zhong Fu - Central Treasury	Jung Bu Chu Fu	Chest, 1 unit below lateral end of clavicle, in first intercostal space, 6 units lateral to CO (pulse).	Intermediate supraclavicular nerve, branches of anterior thoracic nerve and first intercostal nerve, (a pulse can be felt at this point).
LU-2	Yun Men - Cloud Gate	Un Mun Um Mon	Chest, in recess directly below lateral end of clavicle, 6 units lateral to CO, where pulse is felt.	Intermediate+lateral supraclavicular nerve, branches of anterior thoracic nerve, lateral cord of brachial plexus, cephalic vein, thoracoacromial artery and vein.
LU-3	Tian Fu - Celestial Storehouse	Cheon Bu Tem Pu	Upper arm, 3 units below end of axillary fold, at radial side of biceps muscle, 6 units above LU-5.	Lateral brachial cutaneous nerve at point where musculocutaneous nerve passes through; cephalic vein; muscular branches of brachial artery and vein.
LU-4	Xia Bai - Guarding White	Hyeob Baeg Kyo Haku	Upper arm, 1 unit below LU-3, at radial side of biceps brachii muscle, where pulse is felt.	See LU-3.
• LU-5	Chi Ze - Cubit Marsh	Cheog Taeg Shaku Taku	Crease of elbow, at radial side of biceps tendon, at origin of brachioradialis muscle.	Lateral antebrachial cutaneous nerve, radial nerve, branches of radial recurrent artery and vein, cephalic vein.
• LU-6	Kong Zui - Collection Hole	Gong Choe Ko Sai	Thumb-side of arm, midway between wrist and elbow, 5 units below LU-5, 7 units above LU-9.	Lateral antebrachial cutaneous nerve, superficial branch of radial nerve, radial artery and vein, cephalic vein.
• LU-7	Lie Que - Broken Sequence	Yeol Gyeol Retsu Ketsu	Thumb-side of forearm, in crevice at lateral edge of radius bone, 1.5 units above wrist crease.	Lateral antebrachial cutaneous nerve, superficial branch of radial nerve, radial artery, cephalic vein.
• LU-8	Jing Qu - Channel Ditch	Gyeong Geo Kei Kyo	Wrist at palmar crease, 1 unit above transverse crease, in recess on radial side of radial artery.	Lateral antebrachial cutaneous nerve, superficial branch of radial nerve.
LU-9	Tai Yuan - Great Abyss	Tae Yeon Dai En	Wrist at transverse crease, in recess on radial side of radial artery, where pulse is felt.	Lateral antebrachial cutaneous nerve, superficial branch of radial nerve, radial artery and vein.
• LU-10	Yu Ji - Fish Border	Eo Je Gyo Sai	On thenar eminence between red skin (palm) and white skin (back hand), middle of 1st metacarpal.	Superficial branch of radial nerve, venules of thumb draining to cephalic vein, (thenar eminence is the "fleshy bulge below thumb").
LU-11	Shao Shang - Lesser Shang	So Sang Sho Sho	Radial side of thumb, about 0.1 unit proximal to (above) corner of nail.	Terminal nerve network formed by mixed branches of lateral antebrachial cutaneous nerve, superior branch of radial nerve, and palmar digital proprial nerve of median n.

Large Intestine (LI)

Primary Paths

The Large Intestine meridian begins externally, at the radial side of the forefinger (LI-1). It ascends the outside of the arm, passes over the shoulder joint and intersects SI-12, then GV-14. It then enters the body at the supra-clavicular fossa, and travels straight to ST-12. Here it divides into two branches: one internal and one external. The internal branch connects with the Lung, descends through the diaphragm, and enters its home Organ, the Large Intestine. The external branch ascends the front of the neck, crosses the cheek and enters the lower gum. From here, it travels externally across the upper lip, ending at the far side of the nostril (LI-20). Note that the left and right Large Intestine meridians cross each other at the philtrum.

Function

Large Intestine acupoints influence the face, eyes, ears, nose, gums, teeth, throat, skin and intestines; and relate to fever diseases, water metabolism and the elimination of water.

Key Data

Type:	Yang
Phase:	Metal
Acupoints:	20 (x2)
Qi-Flow:	5 am – 7 am
Connects with:	Lung
Communication:	Stomach

Special Points

Source-Yuan:	LI-4
Connecting-Luo:	LI-6
Cleft-Xi:	LI-7
Alarm-Mu:	ST-25
Associated-Shu:	BL-25
Lower Uniting:	ST-37
Command (face):	LI-4

Intersection-Jiaohui Points

Yang Heel — LI-15, 16

Points intersecting Large Intestine:
GV-14, 26
SI-12
ST-4, 12, 37
TW-20

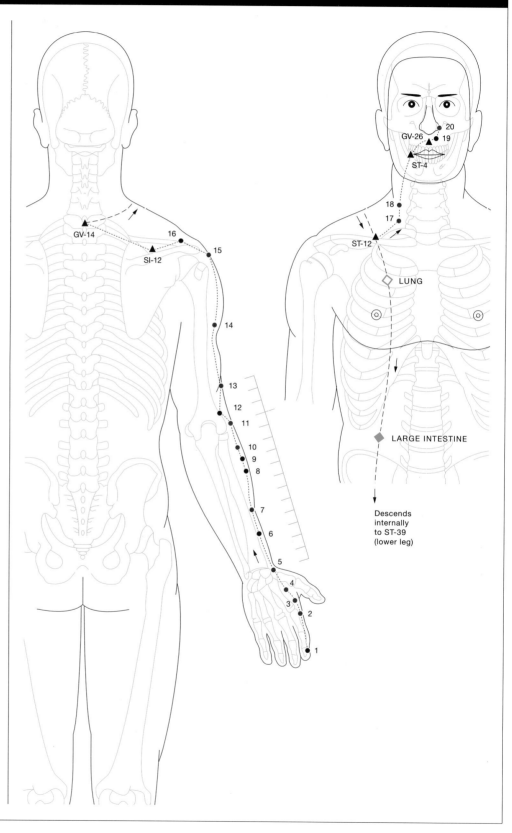

Large Intestine (LI)

Symbol	Chinese Name	Korean Japanese	Location	Local Anatomy (Nerves and Blood Vessels)
LI-1	Shang Yang - Shang Yang	Sang Yang Sho Yo	Radial side of index finger, about 0.1 unit proximal to (above) corner of nail.	Palmar digital propial nerve of median nerve, the arterial-venous network formed by the dorsal and digital arteries and veins.
• LI-2	Er Jian - Second Space	I Gan Ji Kan	Radial side of index finger, distal to metacarpo-phalangeal joint, between red and white skin.	Dorsal digital nerve of radial nerve, palmar digital propial nerve of median nerve, dorsal digital and palmar digital propial arteries and veins (from radial artery + vein).
• LI-3	San Jian - Third Space	Sam Gan San Kan	Radial side of index finger, proximal to head of second metacarpal bone, in recess at base joint.	Superficial branch of radial nerve, dorsal venous network of hand, branch of first dorsal metacarpal artery.
• LI-4	He Gu - Union Valley	Hab Gog Go Koku	Center of muscle between 1st + 2nd metacarpals on back of hand (web of thumb), slightly to 2nd.	Superficial branch of radial nerve, palmar digital propial nerve of median nerve (located deeper).
• LI-5	Yang Xi - Yang Ravine	Yang Gye Yo Kei	Radial side of wrist, in recess between extensor muscle tendons at base of thumb.	Superficial branch of radial nerve, radial artery, dorsal carpal branch of radial artery, cephalic vein.
LI-6	Pian Li - Veering Passage	Pyeon Leog Hen Reki	3 units above the wrist and LI-5, 1/4 of the distance on a line joining LI-5 to LI-11.	Cephalic vein. On radial side: lateral antebrachial cutaneous n. and superficial branch of radial nerve. On ulnar side, posterior cutaneous n. and posterior interosseous n.
• LI-7	Wen Liu - Warm Flow	On Ryu On Ru	Thumb-side of forearm, 5 units above LI-5, 2 units above LI-6.	Posterior antebrachial cutaneous nerve, deep branch of radial nerve, muscular branch of radial artery, cephalic vein.
LI-8	Xia Lian - Lower Ridge	Ha Ryeom Ge Ren	Thumb-side of forearm, 4 units below LI-11, at edge of bulging flesh along radius bone.	See LI-7.
LI-9	Shang Lian - Upper Ridge	Sang Ryeom Jo Ren	Thumb-side of forearm, 1 unit above LI-8, 3 units below LI-11, on a line joining LI-5 to LI-11.	See LI-7.
• LI-10	Shou San Li - Arm Three Li	Su Sam Ri Te San Ri	Thumb-side of forearm, 2 units below elbow, 2 units below LI-11 (flesh bulges when pressed).	Nerves as listed under LI-7, branches of radial recurrent artery and vein.
• LI-11	Qu Chi - Pool at the Bend	Gog Ji Kyoku Chi	In recess at lateral end of elbow crease, midway between LU-5 and protruding humerus bone .	Posterior antebrachial cutaneous nerve, radial nerve (located deeper on medial side), branches of radial recurrent artery and vein.
LI-12	Zhou Liao - Elbow Bone-Hole	Ju Ryo Chu Ryo	Recess above protruding humerus bone at outer elbow (when bent), 1 unit above+lateral to LI-11.	Posterior antebrachial cutaneous nerve, radial nerve (located deeper on medial side), radial collateral artery and vein.
• LI-13	(Shou) Wu Li - (Arm) Five Li	(Su) O Ri (Te) Go Ri	In recess near edge of biceps, 3 units above LI-11 on a line joining LI-11 to LI-15 (pulse felt).	Posterior antebrachial cutaneous nerve, radial nerve (located deeper), radial collateral artery and vein.
• LI-14	Bi Nao - Upper Arm	Bi No Hi Ju	Upper arm, slightly above deltoid muscle insertion at bone, on line joining LI-11 to LI-15.	Posterior brachial cutaneous nerve, radial nerve (located deeper), branches of posterior circumflex humeral artery and vein, deep brachial artery and vein.
• LI-15	Jian Yu - Shoulder Bone	Gyeon U Ken Gu	With arm raised, in a recess at edge of shoulder joint, slightly forward to middle of deltoid muscle.	Axillary nerve, lateral supraclavicular nerve, posterior circumflex humeral artery and vein.
LI-16	Ju Gu - Great Bone	Geo Gol Ko Kotsu	Top of shoulder, in recess between end of clavicle and scapular spine (between 2 forking bones).	Lateral supraclavicular nerve and branch of accessory nerve (near surface), suprascapular nerve (deeper), jugular vein, suprascapular artery and vein (deeper).
• LI-17	Tian Ding - Celestial Tripod	Cheon Jeong Ten Tei	In a recess at the side of base of neck, on rear edge of sternoceidomastoid muscle .	Supraclavicular nerve where cutaneous cervical nerve emerges, phrenic nerve (deeper), external jugular vein.
• LI-18	Fu Tu - Protuberance Assistant	Bu Dol Fu Totsu	Side of neck, level with Adam's apple tip, directly below ear, on rear part of sternoceidomastoid m.	Great auricular nerve, cutaneous cervical nerve, lesser occipital nerve, accessory nerve, ascending cervical artery and vein (deeper on medial side).
LI-19	He Liao - Grain Bone-Hole	Wha Ryo Ka Ryo	Directly below lateral edge of nostril, level with GV-26 at philtrum (upper lip).	Anastomotic branch of facial and infraorbital nerves, superior labial branches of facial artery and vein.
• LI-20	Ying Xiang - Welcome Fragrance	Yeong Hyang Gei Ko	Side of nose, in nasolabial groove, level with midpoint of ala nasi (bulge), 1 unit from LI-19.	Anastomotic branch of facial and infraorbital nerves, facial artery and vein, infraorbital artery and vein.

Stomach (ST)

Primary Paths

The Stomach meridian begins internally, at the side of the nostril, at the point where the Large Intestine meridian ends (LI-20). It ascends to the inner corner of the eye, intersecting BL-1. It emerges below the eye (ST-1), descends along the side of the nose, enters the upper gum, and intersects GV-26 on the upper lip. From here, it descends to the chin, intersecting CO-24; circles up the side of the face, intersecting GB-3, GB-4 and GB-6; and traverses to the middle of the forehead, intersecting GV-24.

An external branch separates at the jaw, descends along the neck, enters the body, and crosses through to the upper back, intersecting GV-14. From here, it descends across the diaphragm, intersecting CO-13 and CO-12. It then enters its home Organ, the Stomach, and connects with the Spleen.

Another external branch descends from the supraclavicular fossa (ST-12), down over the chest and abdomen, ending in the groin (ST-30).

Internally, another branch begins in the lower end of the stomach (pylorus), and descends to the groin, connecting with the external path at ST-30. From here, it descends externally along the leg, ending at the outer corner of the second toenail (ST-45).

Two more internal branches are found on the lower leg: the first branches from the main meridian, at ST-36 (below the knee), and ends at the lateral side of the middle toe; the second branches from ST-42 (top of foot), and ends at the medial side of big toe, where it connects with the Spleen meridian at SP-1.

Function

Stomach acupoints influence the face, nose, gums, throat, stomach, intestines, and general mental states, and relate to fever diseases.

Key Data

Type:	Yang
Phase:	Earth
Acupoints:	45 (x2)
Qi-Flow:	7 am – 9 am
Connects with:	Spleen
Communication:	Large Intestine

Special Points

Source-Yuan:	ST-42
Connecting-Luo:	ST-40
Cleft-Xi:	ST-34
Alarm-Mu:	CO-12
Associated-Shu:	BL-21
Lower Uniting:	ST-36

Intersection-Jiaohui Points

Large Intestine —	ST-4, 12, 37
Small Intestine —	ST-39
Gallbladder —	ST-5, 7, 8, 12
Conception ---	ST-1
Penetrating ---	ST-30
Yang Heel —	ST-1, 3, 4

Points intersecting Stomach:
BL-1
CO-12, 13, 24
GB-3, 4, 6
GV-14, 24, 26

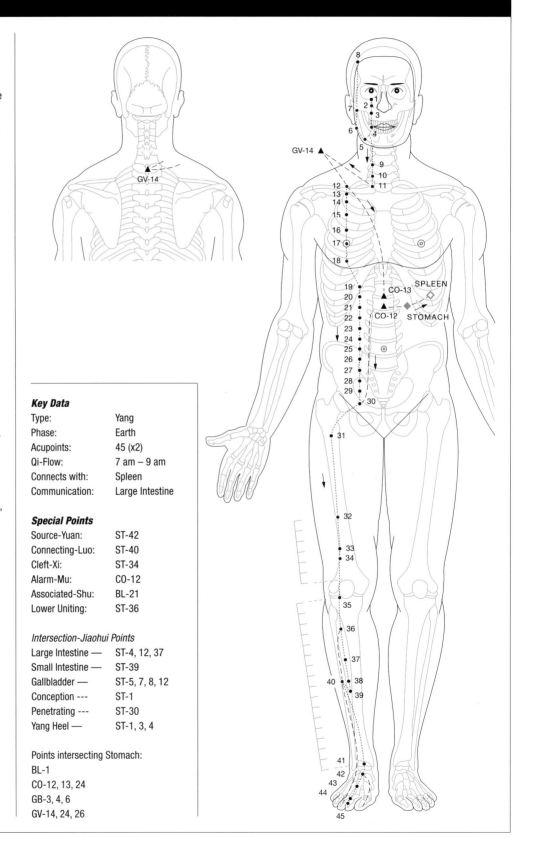

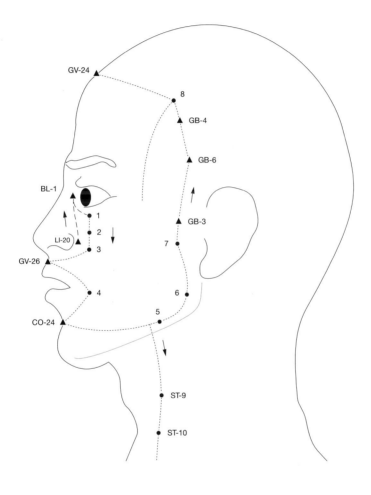

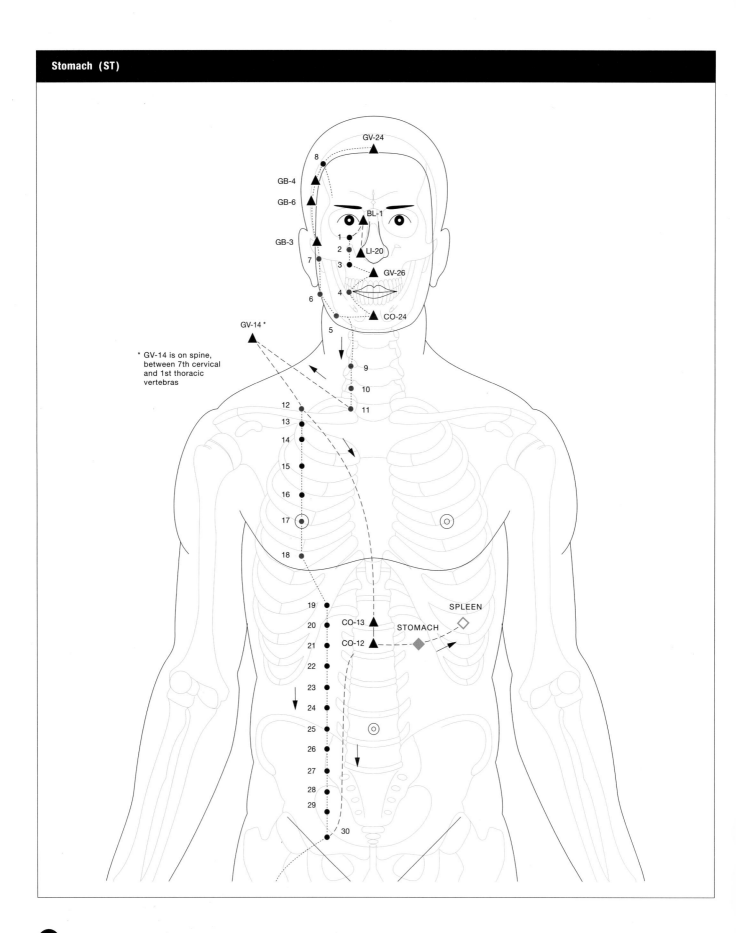

GV-24
8
GB-4
GB-6
BL-1
1
2
LI-20
GB-3
3
7
GV-26
6
4
CO-24
GV-14 *
5
* GV-14 is on spine,
between 7th cervical
and 1st thoracic
vertebras
9
10
12
11
13
14
15
16
17
18
19
20
CO-13
SPLEEN
21
CO-12
STOMACH
22
23
24
25
26
27
28
29
30

Stomach (ST)

Symbol	Chinese Name	Korean / Japanese	Location	Local Anatomy (Nerves and Blood Vessels)
ST-1	Cheng Qi - Tear Container	Seung Eub / Sho Kyu	Directly below eye pupil, in recess above cheekbone at lower eyelid.	Branch of intraorbital nerve, inferior branch of oculomotor nerve, muscular branch of facial nerve, branches of infraorbital and ophthalmic arteries and veins.
• ST-2	Si Bai - Four Whites	Sa Baeg / Shi Haku	In a recess on top edge of cheekbone, aligned with eye pupil and ST-1.	Point lies exactly on the infraorbital nerve. Branches of facial artery and vein, infraorbital artery and vein
ST-3	Ju Liao - Great Bone-Hole	Geo Ryo / Ko Ryo	Directly below eye pupil and ST-1 and ST-2, level with lower edge of nostril.	Branches of facial and infraorbital nerves, branches of facial and infraorbital arteries and veins.
• ST-4	Di Cang - Earth Granary	Ji Chang / Chi So	Slightly lateral to corner of mouth, directly below ST-3, a faint pulse is felt close below.	Branches of facial and infraorbital nerves, terminal branch of buccal nerve (deeper), facial and artery and vein.
• ST-5	Da Ying - Great Reception	Dae Yeong / Dai Gei	In a groove-like recess along bottom of jaw bone, on front edge of masseter muscle (pulse is felt).	Facial and buccal nerves, facial artery and vein.
• ST-6	Jia Che - Jawbone	Hyeob Geo / Kyo Sha	0.75 unit above and forward to lower angle of mandible, at masseter m. bulge (teeth clenched).	At point where masseter muscle attaches. Great auricular nerve, facial nerve, masseteric nerve.
• ST-7	Xia Guan - Below the Joint	Ha Gwan / Ge Kan	In front of ear, in recess at lower edge of zygomatic arch, forward of jaw joint.	Zygomatic branch of facial nerve, branch of auriculotemporal nerve, transverse facial artery and vein, maxillary artery and vein (deeper).
ST-8	Tou Wei - Head Corner	Du Yu / Zul	At corner of forehead, 0.5 unit within hairline, 4.5 units lateral to Governing meridian.	Branch of auriculotemporal nerve and temporal branch of facial nerve. Frontal branches of superficial temporal artery and vein.
• ST-9	Ren Ying - Man's Prognosis	In Yeong / Jin Gei	Side of neck, level with Adam's apple tip, at front edge of sternocleidomastoid m., along carotid a.	Cutaneous cervical nerve, cervical branch of facial nerve, branch of hypoglossal and vagus nerves, point where carotid artery branches, thyroid artery, anterior jugular v.
• ST-10	Shui Tu - Water Prominence	Su Dol / Sui Totsu	On front edge of sternocleidomastoid muscle, halfway between ST-9 and ST-11.	Cutaneous cervical nerve (near surface), superior cardiac nerve branching from sympathetic nerve and trunk (deeper), common carotid artery.
• ST-11	Qi She - Qi Abode	Gi Sa / Ki Sha	Front base of neck, in recess between two heads of sternocleidomastoid m., at end of clavicle.	Medial supraclavicular nerve, muscular branch of ansa hypoglossi, anterior jugular vein (near surface), common carotid artery (deeper).
• ST-12	Que Pen - Empty Basin	Gyeol Bun / Ketsu Bon	In a recess at top edge of middle of clavicle, aligned with nipple, 4 units lateral to midline.	Intermediate supraclavicular nerve (near surface), supraclavicular part of brachial plexus (deeper), transverse cervical artery.
ST-13	Qi Hu - Qi Door	Gi Ho / Ki Ko	In a recess at lower edge of middle of clavicle, above and aligned with nipple.	Branches of supraclavicular nerve and anterior thoracic nerve, branches of thoracoacromial artery and vein, subclavicular vein.
ST-14	Ku Fang - Storeroom	Go Bang / Ko Bo	Chest, in 1st intercostal space (between ribs), above and aligned with nipple.	Branch of anterior thoracic nerve, thoracoacromial artery and vein, branches of lateral thoracic artery and vein.
ST-15	Wu Yi - Roof	Og Ye / Oku Ei	Chest, in 2nd intercostal space (between ribs), above and aligned with nipple.	Anterior cutaneous branches of thoracic nerves, medial pectoral nerve, pectoral branch of thoracoacromial artery and vein, 2nd intercostal artery and vein.
ST-16	Ying Chuang - Breast Window	Eung Chang / Yo So	Chest, in 3rd intercostal space (between ribs), above and aligned with nipple.	Branch of anterior thoracic nerve, lateral thoracic artery and vein.
• ST-17	Ru Zhong - Breast Center	Yu Jung / Nyu Chu	Chest, in center of nipple. This acupoint is often used as a landmark to locate other acupoints.	Anterior and lateral cutaneous branches of 4th intercostal nerve.
• ST-18	Ru Gen - Breast Root	Yu Geun / Nyu Kon	Chest, in 5th intercostal space (between ribs), one rib below nipple, aligned with nipple.	Branch of 5th intercostal nerve, branches of intercostal artery and vein.
ST-19	Bu Rong - Not Contained	Bul Yong / Fu Yo	Abdomen, 6 units above navel, 2 units lateral to CO-14.	Branch of 7th intercostal nerve, branches of 7th intercostal and superior epigastric arteries and veins.
ST-20	Cheng Man - Assuming Fullness	Seung Man / Sho Man	Abdomen, 5 units above navel, 2 units lateral to CO-13, 1 unit below ST-19.	See ST-19.
ST-21	Liang Men - Beam Gate	Yang Mun / Ryo Mon	Abdomen, 4 units above navel, 2 units lateral to CO-12, 1 unit below ST-20.	Branches of 8th intercostal and superior epigastric arteries and veins.
ST-22	Guan Men - Pass Gate	Gwan Mun / Kam Mon	Abdomen, 3 units above navel, 2 units lateral to CO-11, 1 unit below ST-21.	See ST-21.
ST-23	Tai Yi - Supreme Unity	Tae Eul / Tai Itsu	Abdomen, 2 units above navel, 2 units lateral to CO-10, 1 unit below ST-22.	Branches of 8th and 9th intercostal nerves, branches of 8th and 9th intercostal and inferior epigastric arteries and veins.

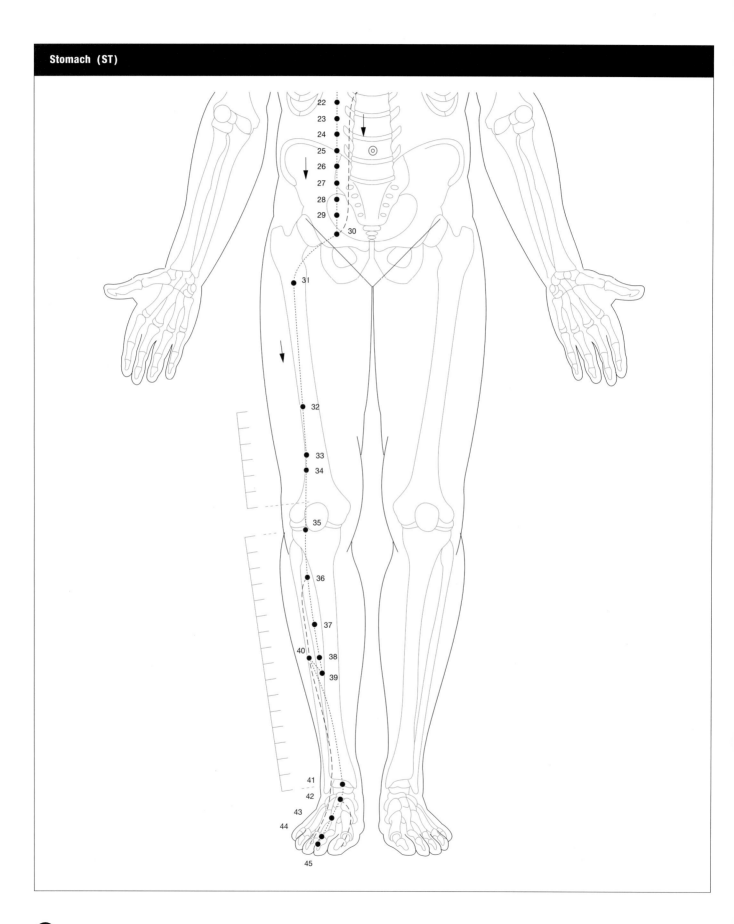

Symbol	Chinese Name	Korean Japanese	Location	Local Anatomy (Nerves and Blood Vessels)
ST-24	Hua Rou Men - Slippery Flesh Gate	Hwal Yug Mun Katsu Niku Mon	Abdomen, 1 unit above navel, 2 units lateral to CO-9, 1 unit below ST-23.	Branch of 9th intercostal nerve, branches of 9th intercostal and inferior epigastric arteries and veins.
ST-25	Tian Shu - Celestial Pivot	Cheon Chu Ten Su	Abdomen, 2 units lateral to center of navel (CO-8).	Branches of 10th intercostal and inferior epigastric arteries and veins.
ST-26	Wai Ling - Outer Mound	Oe Leung Ge Ryo	Abdomen, 1 unit below navel, 2 units lateral to CO-7, 1 unit below ST-25.	See ST-25.
ST-27	Da Ju - Great Gigantic	Dae Geo Tai Ko	Abdomen, 2 units below navel, 2 units lateral to CO-5, 1 unit below ST-26.	11th intercostal nerve, branches of intercostal artery and vein, inferior epigastric artery and vein (slightly lateral).
ST-28	Shui Dao - Waterway	Su Do Sui Do	Abdomen, 3 units below navel, 2 units lateral to CO-4, 1 unit below ST-27.	Branch of subcostal nerve, branches subcostal artery and vein, inferior epigastric artery and vein (slightly lateral).
ST-29	Gui Lai - Return	Gwi Rae Ki Rai	Abdomen, 4 units below navel, 2 units lateral to CO-3, 1 unit below ST-28.	Iliohypogastric nerve, inferior epigastric artery and vein (slightly lateral).
ST-30	Qi Chong - Surging Qi	Gi Chung Ki Sho	5 units below navel, 2 units lateral to CO-2, above inguinal groove, medial side of femoral a.	Path of Ilioinguinal nerve, branches of superficial epigastric artery and vein, inferior epigastric artery and vein (slightly lateral), femoral artery (pulse is felt).
ST-31	Bi Guan - Inferior Joint	Bi Gwan Hi Kan	Thigh, in recess on lateral side of sartorius muscle (thigh flexed), level with perineum.*	Lateral femoral cutaneous nerve, branches of lateral circumflex femoral artery and vein (deeper). *Note: ST-31 is below + aligned with front-upper iliac spine of hipbone.
• ST-32	Fu Tu - Crouching Rabbit	Bog To Fuku To	Thigh, 6 units above top lateral edge of kneecap, in middle of belly of rectus femoris muscle.	Anterior and lateral femoral cutaneous nerves, branches of lateral circumflex femoral artery and vein.
ST-33	Yin Shi - Yin Market	Eum Si In Shi	Thigh, 3 units above top lateral edge of kneecap, between rectus femoris and vastus lateralis m.	Anterior and lateral femoral cutaneous nerves, descending branch of lateral circumflex femoral artery.
• ST-34	Liang Qiu - Beam Hill	Yang Gu Ryo Kyu	Thigh, 2 units above top lateral edge of kneecap, between rectus femoris and vastus lateralis m.	See ST-33.
• ST-35	Du Bi - Calf's Nose	Dog Bi Toku Bi	In a recess below kneecap, lateral to patellar ligament when knee is bent.	Lateral sural cutaneous nerve, articular branch of common peroneal nerve, arterial and venous network around the knee joint.
• ST-36	Zu San Li - Leg Three Li	Jog Sam Ri Ashi San Ri	Lower leg, 3 units below ST-35, about 1 unit lateral to crest of tibia bone (shinbone).	Lateral sural cutaneous nerve and cutaneous branch of saphenous nerve (near surface), deep peroneal nerve (deeper), anterior tibial artery and vein.
ST-37	Shang Ju Xu - Upper Great Hollow	Sang Ryeom Jo Ko Kyo	Lower leg, 6 units below ST-35, about 0.75 unit lateral to front crest of tibia bone (shinbone).	See ST-36.
ST-38	Tiao Kou - Ribbon Opening	Jo Gu Jo Ko	Leg, 2 units below ST-37, 8 units below ST-35, midway between ST-35 + 41, near edge of tibia.	See ST-36.
ST-39	Xia Ju Xu - Lower Great Hollow	Ha Ryeom Ge Ko Kyo	Lower leg, 0.75 unit lateral to front crest of tibia, 3 units below ST-37, 9 units below knee (ST-35).	Branches of superficial peroneal and deep peroneal nerves, anterior tibial artery and vein.
• ST-40	Feng Long - Bountiful Bulge	Pung Ryung Ho Ryu	Lower leg, about 0.75 unit lateral to ST-38, 8 units below ST-35, 8 units above ankle.	Superficial peroneal nerve, branches of anterior tibial artery and vein.
ST-41	Jie Xi - Ravine Divide	Hae Gye Kai Kei	Ankle joint, between extensor muscle tendons of toes and big toe, level to outer protruding bone.	Superficial peroneal and deep peroneal nerves, anterior tibial artery and vein.
ST-42	Chong Yang - Surging Yang	Chung Yang Sho Yo	Highest point on top surface of foot, in recess between 2nd+3rd metatarsal+cuneiform bones.	Medial dorsal cutaneous nerve from superficial peroneal nerve (near surface), deep peroneal nerve (deeper), dorsal artery and vein, venous network of foot.
ST-43	Xian Gu - Sunken Valley	Ham Gog Kan Koku	Top of foot, in a recess below (distal) junction of 2nd and 3rd metatarsal bones.	Medial dorsal cutaneous nerve of foot, dorsal venous network of foot.
ST-44	Nei Ting - Inner Court	Nae Jeong Nai Tei	Between 2nd + 3rd toes, in recess below (distal) and lateral to 2nd metatarsophalangeal joint.	Point where lateral branch of medial dorsal cutaneous nerve branches into the dorsal digital nerves, dorsal venous network of foot.
ST-45	Li Dui - Severe Mouth	Yeo Tae Rei Da	Lateral side of 2nd toe, about 0.1 unit above (proximal) to corner of nail.	Dorsal digital nerve of superficial peroneal nerve, arterial and venous network formed by dorsal digital artery and

Spleen (SP)

Primary Paths

The Spleen meridian begins externally, at the top medial tip of big toe (SP-1). It runs along the inside of the foot and ascends the inner leg and abdomen, intersecting the Conception meridian at several points. It then runs internally to enter its home Organ, the Spleen, and connect with the Stomach. The external pathway continues to ascend the abdomen and chest, intersecting GB-24, LV-14 and LU-1. At the chest, it enters the body, ascending the throat to the root of the tongue, under which it disperses Qi. An internal branch separates in the Stomach area, and ascends through the diaphragm, entering the Heart.

Function

Spleen acupoints influence the lips, upper abdomen, stomach, intestines, digestion, and urogenital system.

Key Data

Type:	Yin
Phase:	Earth
Acupoints:	21 (x2)
Qi-Flow:	9 am – 11 am
Connects with:	Stomach
Communication:	Lung

Special Points

Source-Yuan:	SP-3
Connecting-Luo:	SP-4, SP-21
Cleft-Xi:	SP-8
Alarm-Mu:	LV-13
Associated-Shu:	BL-20

Intersection-Jiaohui Points

Kidney ---	SP-6
Liver ---	SP-6, 12, 13
Yin Linking ---	SP-12, 13, 15, 16

Points intersecting Spleen:
CO-3, 4, 10, 17
GB-24
LU-1
LV-14

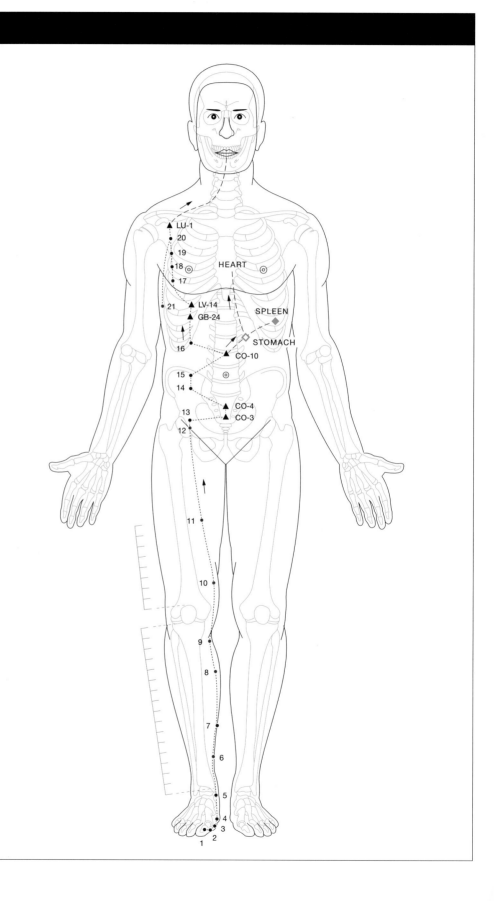

Spleen (SP)

Symbol	Chinese Name	Korean Japanese	Location	Local Anatomy (Nerves and Blood Vessels)
SP-1	Yin Bai - Hidden White	Eun Baeg Im Paku	Medial side of big toe, about 0.1 unit above (proximal) to corner of nail.	On the anastomosis of dorsal digital nerve derived from superficial peroneal nerve and plantar digital proprial nerve, dorsal digital artery.
SP-2	Da Du - Great Metropolis	Dae Do Tai To	Lower medial side of big toe, below (distal) 1st metatarsophalangeal joint, at red+white skin.	Plantar digital proprial nerve derived from medial plantar nerve, branches of medial plantar artery and vein.
SP-3	Tai Bai - Supreme White	Tae Baeg Tai Haku	In recess behind (proximal + inferior) head of metatarsal bone, at edge of red and white skin.	Branches of saphenous nerve and superficial peroneal nerve, medial plantar artery, branches of medial tarsal artery, dorsal venous network of foot.
SP-4	Gong Sun - Yellow Emperor	Gong Son Ko Son	In recess, 1 unit below (distal + inferior) base of 1st metatarsal bone, at edge of red + white skin.	Saphenous nerve, branch of superficial peroneal nerve, medial tarsal artery, dorsal venous network of foot.
SP-5	Shang Qiu - Shang Hill	Sang Gu Sho Kyu	In recess anterior to + slightly below protruding bone at inner ankle, between LV-4 and KI-6.	Medial crural cutaneous nerve, branch of superficial peroneal nerve, medial tarsal artery, great saphenous vein.
• SP-6	San Yin Jiao - Three Yin Intersection	Sam Eum Gyo San In Ko	3 units above protruding bone at inner ankle, on rear (posterior) edge of tibia.	Medial crural cutaneous nerve (near surface), tibial nerve (deeper), great saphenous vein, posterior tibial artery and vein.
SP-7	Lou Gu - Leaking Valley	Nu Gog Ro Koku	6 units above protruding bone at inner ankle, 3 units above SP-6.	See SP-6.
• SP-8	Di Ji - Earth's Crux	Ji Gi Chi Ki	3 units below protruding tibia bone at inner knee, on line joining SP-9 and protruding anklebone.	Medial crural cutaneous nerve, tibial nerve (deeper), great saphenous vein and branch of genu suprema artery (slightly anterior), posterior tibial artery and vein (deeper).
• SP-9	Yin Ling Quan - Yin Mound Spring	Eum Leung Cheon In Ryo Sen	In recess below protruding tibia at inner knee, between rear edge of tibia and gastrocnemius m.	See SP-8. Note: SP-9 is at end of crease when knee is bent.
• SP-10	Xue Hai - Sea of Blood	Hyeol Hae Kekkai	Thigh, 2 units above top medial edge of kneecap, on medial edge of vastus medialis m. (on bulge).	Anterior femoral cutaneous nerve, muscular branch of femoral nerve, muscular branch of femoral artery and vein.
• SP-11	Ji Men - Winnower Gate	Gi Mun Ki Mon	Thigh, 6 units above SP-10, at medial side of sartorius m., between SP-10 + 12 (pulse is felt).	Anterior femoral cutaneous nerve, saphenous nerve (deeper), great saphenous vein, femoral artery and vein (deeper and lateral).
• SP-12	Chong Men - Surging Gate	Chung Mun Sho Mon	In inguinal crease, lateral side of femoral artery, 3.5 units lateral to CO-2, where pulse is felt.	Point where femoral nerve traverses, femoral artery (on medial side).
SP-13	Fu She - Bowel Abode	Bu Sa Fu Sha	Abdomen, 0.7 unit above SP-12, 3.5 units lateral to body midline.	Ilioinguinal nerve.
SP-14	Fu Jie - Abdominal Bind	Bog Gyeol Fuku Ketsu	Abdomen, 3 units above SP-13, 1.3 units below SP-15, on lateral side of rectus abdominus m.	11th intercostal nerve, 11th intercostal artery and vein.
SP-15	Da Heng - Great Horizontal	Dae Hoeng Dai O	Abdomen, 3.5 units lateral to center of navel, at lateral edge of rectus abdominus muscle.	10th intercostal nerve, 10th intercostal artery and vein.
SP-16	Fu Ai - Abdominal Lament	Bog Ae Fuku Ai	Abdomen, 3 units above SP-15, 3.5 units lateral to body midline.	8th intercostal nerve, 8th intercostal artery and vein.
SP-17	Shi Dou - Food Hole	Sig Du Shoku Toku	Chest, in 5th intercostal space, 6 units lateral to midline, 2 units lateral to nipple line.	Lateral cutaneous branch of 5th intercostal nerve, thoracoepigastric vein.
SP-18	Tian Xi - Celestial Ravine	Cheon Gye Ten Kei	Chest, in 4th intercostal space (between ribs), 2 units lateral to nipple.	Lateral cutaneous branch of 4th intercostal nerve, thoracoepigastric artery and vein, 4th intercostal artery and vein, branches of lateral thoracic artery and vein.
SP-19	Xiong Xiang - Chest Village	Hyung Hyang Kyo Kyo	Chest, in 3rd intercostal space (between ribs), above SP-18, 6 units lateral to body midline.	Lateral cutaneous branch of 3rd intercostal nerve, 3rd intercostal artery and vein, lateral thoracic artery and vein.
SP-20	Zhou Rong - All-Round Flourishing	Ju Yeong Shu Ei	Chest, in 2nd intercostal space, above SP-19, below LU-1, 6 units lateral to midline.	Muscular branch of anterior thoracic nerve, lateral cutaneous branch of 2nd intercostal nerve, lateral thoracic artery and vein, 2nd intercostal artery and vein.
• SP-21	Da Bao - Great Embracement	Dae Po Tai Ho	Trunk, on midaxillary line, 6 units below armpit, halfway between armpit and free end of 11th rib.	7th intercostal nerve, terminal branch of long thoracic nerve, 7th intercostal artery and vein, thoracodorsal artery and vein.

Heart (HT)

Primary Paths

The Heart meridian has three primary paths, all of which originate in the Heart. The first path emerges through the blood vessel network encircling the Heart, descends internally, through the diaphragm, and connects with the Small Intestine. The second path ascends internally, alongside the throat (esophagus), enters the tissue behind the eye, and connects with the Brain. The third path travels lateral from the Heart to enter the Lung, then slopes downward, emerging in the armpit at HT-1. From here, it descends externally, along the inner arm and palm, ending at the inner edge of the little finger, near the corner of the fingernail (HT-9).

Function

Heart acupoints influence the tongue, chest, heart, blood vessels and general mental states.

Key Data

Type:	Yin
Phase:	Fire
Acupoints:	9 (x2)
Qi-Flow:	11 am – 1 pm
Connects with:	Small Intestine
Communication:	Kidney

Special Points

Source-Yuan:	HT-7
Connecting-Luo:	HT-5
Cleft-Xi:	HT-6
Alarm-Mu:	CO-14
Associated-Shu:	BL-15

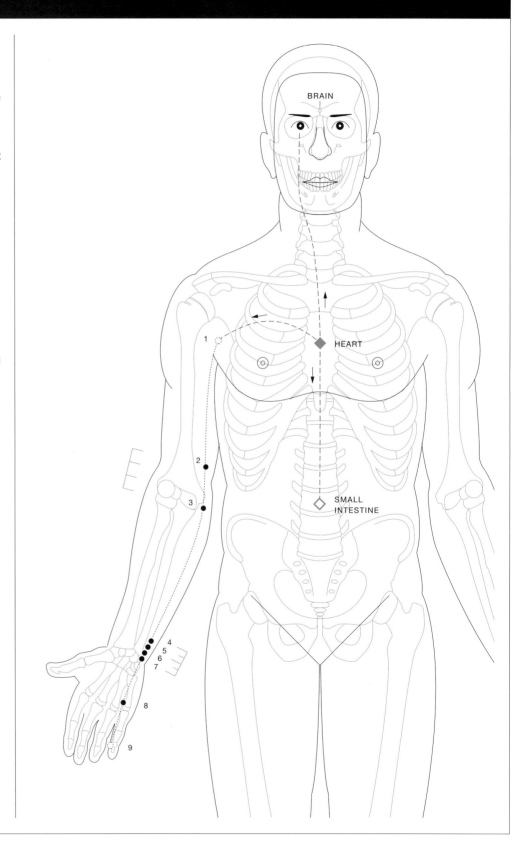

Heart (HT)

Symbol	Chinese Name	Korean Japanese	Location	Local Anatomy (Nerves and Blood Vessels)
• HT-1	Ji Quan - Highest Spring	Geug Cheon Kyoku Sen	With arm raised, in center of axilla (armpit), on medial side of axillary artery.	Ulnar nerve, median nerve, medial brachial cutaneous nerve, Axillary artery (slightly lateral).
• HT-2	Qing Ling - Cyan Spirit	Cheong Lyong Sei Rei	3 units above medial end of elbow crease and HT-3, in groove medial to biceps muscle.	Ulnar nerve, medial antebrachial cutaneous nerve, medial brachial cutaneous nerve, basilic vein, superior ulnar collateral artery.
• HT-3	Shao Hai - Lesser Sea	So Hae Sho Kai	With elbow bent, at medial end of elbow crease, in recess anterior to protruding bone at elbow.	Medial antebrachial cutaneous nerve, basilic vein, inferior ulnar collateral artery, ulnar recurrent artery and vein.
• HT-4	Ling Dao - Spirit Pathway	Yeong Do Rei Do	Forearm, 1.5 units above (proximal) transverse wrist crease, on radial side of flexor tendon.*	Medial antebrachial cutaneous nerve, ulnar nerve (on ulnar side), ulnar artery (*tendon of the flexor carpi ulnaris muscle)
• HT-5	Tong Li - Connecting Li	Tong Ri Tsu Ri	Forearm, 1 unit above (proximal) transverse wrist crease, on radial side of flexor tendon.*	See HT-4. (*tendon of the flexor carpi ulnaris muscle)
• HT-6	Yin Xi - Yin Cleft	Eum Geug In Geki	Forearm, 0.5 unit above (proximal) transverse wrist crease, on radial side of flexor tendon.*	See HT-4. (*tendon of the flexor carpi ulnaris muscle)
• HT-7	Shen Men - Spirit Gate	Sin Mun Shim Mon	On transverse wrist crease, in recess between ulna and pisiform bones, radial side of tendon.*	See HT-4. (*tendon of the flexor carpi ulnaris muscle)
• HT-8	Shao Fu - Lesser Mansion	So Bu Sho Fu	Palm, between 4th and 5th metacarpal bones, above (proximal) metacarpal joint, level to PC-8.	4th common pamar digital nerve derived from ulnar nerve, common palmar digital artery and vein.
HT-9	Shao Chong - Lesser Surge	So Chung Sho Sho	On radial side of little finger, about 0.1 unit proximal to corner of nail.	Pamar digital proprial nerve derived from ulnar nerve, arterial and venous network formed by palmar digital proprial artery and vein.

Small Intestine (SI)

Primary Paths

The Small Intestine meridian begins externally, at the outer edge of the little finger (SI-1). It ascends the outer arm to the back of the shoulder, intersecting BL-11 and BL-36, as it runs to the top-center of the back to intersect GV-14. It then enters the body and divides into two paths: internal and external. The internal branch connects with the Heart, and descends along the esophagus, through the diaphragm, to join the Stomach. It then intersects CO-13 and CO-12, before entering its home Organ, the Small Intestine. The external branch emerges from the body, ascends the side of the neck, circles the cheek (intersecting GB-1 and TW-22), and enters the ear at SI-19. A short branch separates at the cheek and ascends to the inner corner of the eye (BL-1).

Function

Small Intestine acupoints influence the eyes, ears, throat, mental states and the body's regulation of fluids and solids.

Key Data

Type:	Yang
Phase:	Fire
Acupoints:	19 (x2)
Qi-Flow:	1 pm – 3 pm
Connects with:	Heart
Communication:	Bladder

Special Points

Source-Yuan:	SI-4
Connecting-Luo:	SI-7
Cleft-Xi:	SI-6
Alarm-Mu:	CO-4
Associated-Shu:	BL-27
Lower Uniting:	ST-39

Intersection-Jiaohui Points

Large Intestine —	SI-12
Triple Warmer —	SI-12, 18, 19
Gallbladder —	SI-12, 17, 19
Yang Linking —	SI-10
Yang Heel —	SI-10

Points intersecting Small Intestine:

BL-1, 11, 36 [41]	GV-14
CO-12, 13, 17	ST-39
GB-1	TW-22

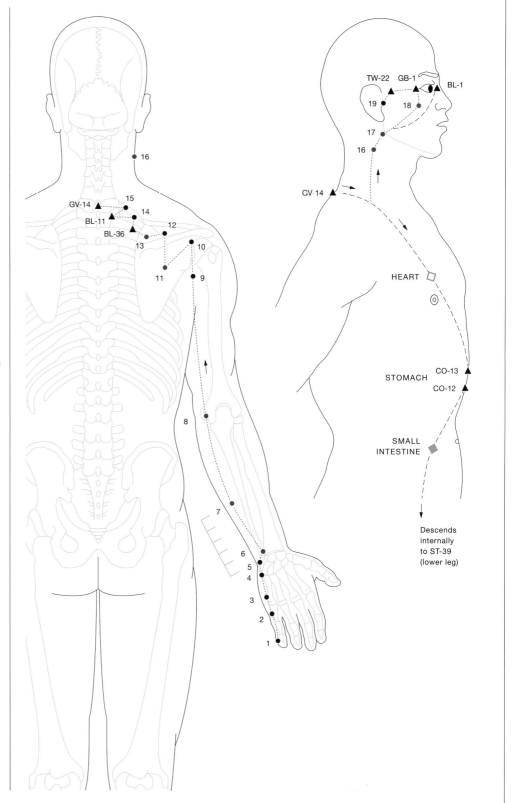

Small Intestine (SI)

Symbol	Chinese Name	Korean Japanese	Location	Local Anatomy (Nerves and Blood Vessels)
SI-1	Shao Ze - Lesser Marsh	So Taeg Sho Taku	On ulnar side of little finger, about 0.1 unit proximal to corner of nail.	Arterial and venous network formed by: palmar digital proprial artery and vein, dorsal digital artery and vein.
SI-2	Qian Gu - Front Valley	Jeon Gog Zen Koku	On ulnar side of little finger, in recess distal (below) metacarpalphalangeal joint.	Dorsal digital nerve, palmar digital proprial nerve from ulnar nerve, dorsal digital artery and vein branching from ulnar artery and vein.
SI-3	Hou Xi - Back Ravine	Hu Gye Go Kei	Ulnar edge of hand, in recess above (proximal and lateral) head of 5th metacarpal bone.	Dorsal branch of ulnar nerve, dorsal artery and vein, dorsal venous network of hand.
SI-4	Wan Gu - Wrist Bone	Wan Gol Wan Kotsu	Ulnar side of hand, in recess between 5th metacarpal bone and triquetral bone of wrist.	Dorsal branch of ulnar nerve, posterior carpal artery (branch of ulnar artery), dorsal venous network of hand.
SI-5	Yang Gu - Yang Valley	Yang Gog Yo Koku	Ulnar side of wrist, in recess between ulna bone and triquetral bone (wrist joint).	Dorsal branch of ulnar nerve, posterior carpal artery.
• SI-6	Yang Lao - Nursing the Aged	Yang Ro Yo Ro	With palm facing chest, 0.5 unit proximal wrist, in bony recess on radial side of head of ulna bone.	Anastomotic branches of posterior antebrachial cutaneous nerve, dorsal branch of ulnar nerve, terminal branches of posterior interosseous artery and vein.
• SI-7	Zhi Zheng - Branch to the Correct	Ji Jeong Shi Sei	Forearm, on medial edge of ulna, 5 units above (proximal) wrist, on line joining SI-5 to SI-8.	Branch of medial antebrachial cutaneous nerve (near surface), posterior interosseous nerve (deeper on radial side), terminal branches of posterior interosseous a. and v.
• SI-8	Xiao Hai - Small Sea	So Hae Sho Kai	In recess on flat spot between elbow point (ulna) and medial bony knob of humerus (arm flexed).	Branches of medial antebrachial cutaneous nerve, ulnar nerve, superior and inferior ulnar collateral arteries and veins, ulnar recurrent artery and vein.
SI-9	Jian Zhen - True Shoulder	Gyeon Jeong Ken Tei	On back, below shoulder joint, 1 unit above end of axillary fold (armpit) when arm is lowered.	Branch of axillary nerve, radial nerve (deeper and above), circumflex scapular artery and vein.
SI-10	Nao Shu - Upper Arm Shu	No Yu Ju Yu	Directly above SI-9 when arm is lowered, in recess below scapular spine (ridge).	Posterior cutaneous nerve of arm, axillary nerve, suprascapular nerve (deeper), posterior circumflex humeral artery and vein, subscapular artery and vein (deeper).
• SI-11	Tian Zong - Celestial Gathering	Cheon Jong Ten So	Flat part of scapula, halfway between left + right edges, 1/3 the distance between ridge and base.	Suprascapular nerve, muscular branches of circumflex scapular artery and vein.
SI-12	Bing Feng - Grasping the Wind	Byeong Pung Hei Fu	Shoulder, above scapular spine (ridge), directly above SI-11, in recess with arm raised.	Lateral subscapular nerve, accessory nerve, suprascapular nerve (deeper), suprascapular artery and vein.
• SI-13	Qu Yuan - Crooked Wall	Gog Weon Kyoku En	Back, halfway between SI-10 and spine, above scapular spine (ridge), in recess at medial end.	Lateral branch of posterior ramus of 2nd thoracic n., accessory n., muscular branch of suprascapular n. (deeper), branches of transverse cervical and suprascapular a. and v.
SI-14	Jian Wai Shu - Outer Shoulder Shu	Gyeon Oe Yu Ken Gai Yu	Upper back, in recess 3 units lateral to GV-13 (T1 vertebra), aligned to medial edge of scapula.	Medial cutaneous branches of posterior ramus of 1st and 2nd thoracic nerves, accessory n., dorsal scapular n. (deeper), transverse cervical artery and vein (deeper).
SI-15	Jian Zhong Shu - Central Shoulder Shu	Gyeon Joong Yu Ken Chu Yu	Upper back, 2 units lateral to spine and GV-14 (7th cervical vertebra), at level of shoulder.	See SI-14.
• SI-16	Tian Chuang - Celestial Window	Cheon Chang Ten So	Side of neck, on rear (posterior) edge of sternocleidomastoid m., above and behind LI-18.	Cutaneous cervical nerve, emerging part of great auricular nerve, ascending cervical artery.
• SI-17	Tian Rong - Celestial Countenance	Cheon Yong Ten Yo	Directly behind corner of jaw (angle of mandible), recess at anterior edge of sternocleidomastoid m.	Anterior branch of great auricular n., cervical branch of facial n., superior cervical ganglion of sympathetic trunk (deeper), carotid and jugular arteries and veins.
• SI-18	Quan Liao - Cheek Bone-Hole	Gwan Ryo Kan Ryo	Below outer corner of eye, in recess below lower edge of protruding cheekbone (zygoma).	Facial and infraorbital nerves, branches of transverse facial artery and vein.
SI-19	Ting Gong - Auditory Palace	Cheong Gung Cho Kyu	Between pearl of ear (tragus) and jaw joint, in recess formed when mouth is wide open.	Branch of facial nerve, auriculotemporal nerve, auricular branches of superficial temporal artery and vein.

Bladder (BL)

Primary Paths

The Bladder meridian begins externally, at the inner corner of the eye (BL-1), and ascends the forehead, intersecting GV-24 and GB-15, as it travels to the vertex of the head (GV-20). At this point, a small branch separates and descends to the area above the ear, intersecting several points on the Gallbladder meridian. Another branch descends vertically from GV-20 into the Brain, and reemerges at GV-17. The exterior path continues to descend the back of the head and neck. There it splits into two parallel lines descending to the buttocks. From here, each line follows eccentric paths, across the buttocks and down the lower leg, crossing before merging near the back of the knee. A single path descends the calf (posterior to anklebone), ending at the lateral tip of the little toe (BL-67).

In the lumbar area, a branch separates and enters the body cavity to connect with the Kidney, before entering its home Organ, the Bladder (see small drawing). The Bladder meridian also joins directly with the Heart.

Function

Bladder acupoints influence the vertex (top of head), eyes, nose, lumbar region, and general mental states, and relate to fever producing diseases.

Key Data

Type:	Yang
Phase:	Water
Acupoints:	67 (x2)
Qi-Flow:	3 pm – 5 pm
Connects with:	Kidney
Communication:	Small Intestine

Special Points

Source-Yuan:	BL-64
Connecting-Luo:	BL-58
Cleft-Xi:	BL-63
Alarm-Mu:	CO-3
Associated-Shu:	BL-28
Lower Uniting:	BL-54
Meeting-Hui (Blood):	BL-17
Meeting-Hui (Bones):	BL-11
Command (Back):	BL-54

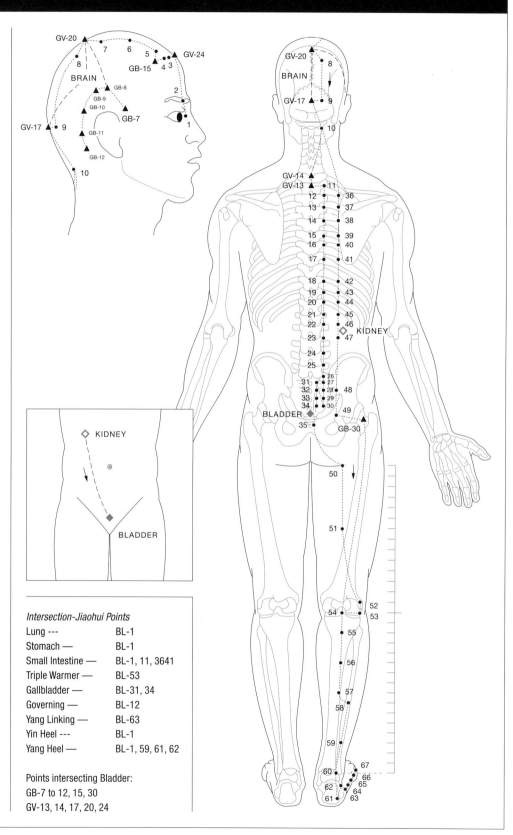

Intersection-Jiaohui Points

Lung ---	BL-1
Stomach —	BL-1
Small Intestine —	BL-1, 11, 3641
Triple Warmer —	BL-53
Gallbladder —	BL-31, 34
Governing —	BL-12
Yang Linking —	BL-63
Yin Heel ---	BL-1
Yang Heel —	BL-1, 59, 61, 62

Points intersecting Bladder:
GB-7 to 12, 15, 30
GV-13, 14, 17, 20, 24

Bladder (BL)

Symbol	Chinese Name	Korean Japanese	Location	Local Anatomy (Nerves and Blood Vessels)
BL-1	Jing Ming - Bright Eyes	Jeong Myeong Sei Mei	0.1 unit above inner corner of eye (inner canthus), located with eyes closed.	Supratrochlear and infratrochlear nerves (near surface), branches of oculomotor nerve (deeper), opthalmic n. (deeper), angular a. and v., opthalmic a. and v. (above, deeper)
BL-2	Zan Zhu - Bamboo Gathering	Chan Jug San Chiku	At inner (medial) end of eyebrow, in recess (supraorbital notch), above BL-1.	Medial branch of frontal nerve, frontal artery and vein.
BL-3	Mei Chong - Eyebrow Ascension	Mi Chung Bi Sho	Head, above BL-2, about 0.5 unit within front hairline, between GV-24 and BL-4.	See BL-2.
BL-4	Qu Chai - Deviating Turn	Gog Cha Kyoku Sa	1.5 units lateral to midline, 0.5 unit within front hairline, 1/3 the distance from GV-24 to ST-8.	Lateral branch of frontal nerve, frontal artery and vein.
BL-5	Wu Chu - Fifth Palace	O Cheo Go Sho	Top of head, behind (posterior) BL-4, 1 unit within front hairline, lateral to GV-23.	See BL-4.
• BL-6	Cheng Guang - Light Guard	Seung Gwang Sho Ko	Top of head, 1.5 units behind (posterior) BL-5, 1.5 units lateral to body midline (GV).	Anastomotic branch of frontal nerve and great occipital nerve, anastomotic network of frontal artery and vein, superficial temporal artery and vein, occipital artery and vein.
• BL-7	Tong Tian - Celestial Connection	Tong Cheon Tsu Ten	Top of head, 1.5 units behind (posterior) BL-6, 1.5 units lateral to body midline (GV).	Branch of great occipital nerve, anastomotic network of superficial temporal artery and vein and occipital artery and vein.
• BL-8	Luo Que - Declining Connection	Nag Geug Rakkyaku	Top of head, 1.5 units behind (posterior) BL-7, 1.5 units lateral to body midline (GV).	Branch of great occipital nerve, branches of occipital artery and vein.
BL-9	Yu Zhen - Jade Pillow	Og Chim Gyoku Chin	Back of head, 1.3 units lateral to GV-17, on lateral upper edge of ext. occipital protuberance.	Occipital artery and vein.
• BL-10	Tian Zhu - Celestial Pillar	Cheon Ju Ten Chu	Back of neck, 1.3 units lateral to GV-15, within hairline, on lateral side of trapezius muscle.	Occipital artery and vein.
BL-11	Da Zhu - Great Shuttle	Dae Jeo Dai Jo	Upper back, 1.5 units lateral to lower edge of spinous process of 1st thoracic vertebra.	Medial cutaneous branches of posterior rami of 1st and 2nd thoracic nerves; deeper, their lateral cutaneous branches, sub-branches of intercostal artery and vein.
BL-12	Feng Men - Wind Gate	Pung Mun Fu Mon	Upper back, 1.5 units lateral to lower edge of spinous process of 2nd thoracic vertebra.	Medial cutaneous branches of posterior rami of 2nd and 3rd thoracic nerves; deeper, their lateral cutaneous branches; sub-branches of intercostal artery and vein.
• BL-13	Fei Shu - Lung Shu	Pye Yu Hai Yu	Upper back, 1.5 units lateral to lower edge of spinous process of 3rd thoracic vertebra.	Medial cutaneous branches of posterior rami of 3rd and 4th thoracic nerves; deeper, their lateral branches; sub-branches of intercostal artery and vein.
• BL-14	Jue Yin Shu - Absolute Yin Shu	Gweol Eum Yu Ketchin Yu	Upper back, 1.5 units lateral to lower edge of spinous process of 4th thoracic vertebra.	Medial cutaneous branches of posterior rami of 4th and 5th thoracic nerves; deeper, their lateral branches; sub-branches of intercostal artery and vein.
• BL-15	Xin Shu - Heart Shu	Sim Yu Shin Yu	Upper back, 1.5 units lateral to lower edge of spinous process of 5th thoracic vertebra.	Medial cutaneous branches of posterior rami of 5th and 6th thoracic nerves; deeper, their lateral branches; sub-branches of intercostal artery and vein.
BL-16	Du Shu - Governing Shu	Dog Yu Toku Yu	Upper back, 1.5 units lateral to lower edge of spinous process of 6th thoracic vertebra.	Dorsal scapular n., medial cutaneous branches of 6th + 7th thoracic nerves; deeper, their lateral branches; branches of intercostal and transverse cervical a. and v.
BL-17	Ge Shu - Diaphragm Shu	Gyeog Yu Kaku Yu	Upper back, 1.5 units lateral to lower edge of spinous process of 7th thoracic vertebra.	Medial cutaneous branches of posterior rami of 7th and 8th thoracic nerves; deeper, their lateral branches; sub-branches of intercostal artery and vein.
BL-18	Gan Shu - Liver Shu	Gan Yu Kan Yu	Back, 1.5 units lateral to lower edge of spinous process of 9th thoracic vertebra.	Medial cutaneous branches of posterior rami of 9th and 10th thoracic nerves; deeper, their lateral branches; sub-branches of intercostal artery and vein.
BL-19	Dan Shu - Gallbladder Shu	Dam Yu Tan Yu	Back, 1.5 units lateral to lower edge of spinous process of 10th thoracic vertebra.	Medial cutaneous branches of posterior rami of 10th and 11th thoracic nerves; deeper, their lateral branches; sub-branches of intercostal artery and vein.
BL-20	Pi Shu - Spleen Shu	Bi Yu Hi Yu	Back, 1.5 units lateral to lower edge of spinous process of 11th thoracic vertebra.	Medial cutaneous branches of posterior rami of 11th and 12th thoracic nerves; deeper, their lateral branches; sub-branches of intercostal artery and vein.
BL-21	Wei Shu - Stomach Shu	Wi Yu I Yu	Back, 1.5 units lateral to lower edge of spinous process of 12th thoracic vertebra.	Medial cutaneous branches of posterior ramus of 12th thoracic nerve; deeper, its lateral branch; sub-branches of intercostal artery and vein.
BL-22	San Jiao Shu - Triple Burner Shu	Sam Cho Yu San Sho Yu	Back, 1.5 units lateral to lower edge of spinous process of 1st lumbar vertebra.	Lateral cutaneous branch of posterior ramus of 10th thoracic nerve; deeper, lateral branch of posterior ramus of 1st lumbar nerve; posterior rami of 1st lumbar a. and v.
• BL-23	Shen Shu - Kidney Shu	Sin Yu Jin Yu	Back, 1.5 units lateral to lower edge of spinous process of 2nd lumbar vertebra.	Branch of posterior ramus of 1st lumbar nerve; posterior ramus of 2nd lumbar artery and vein.

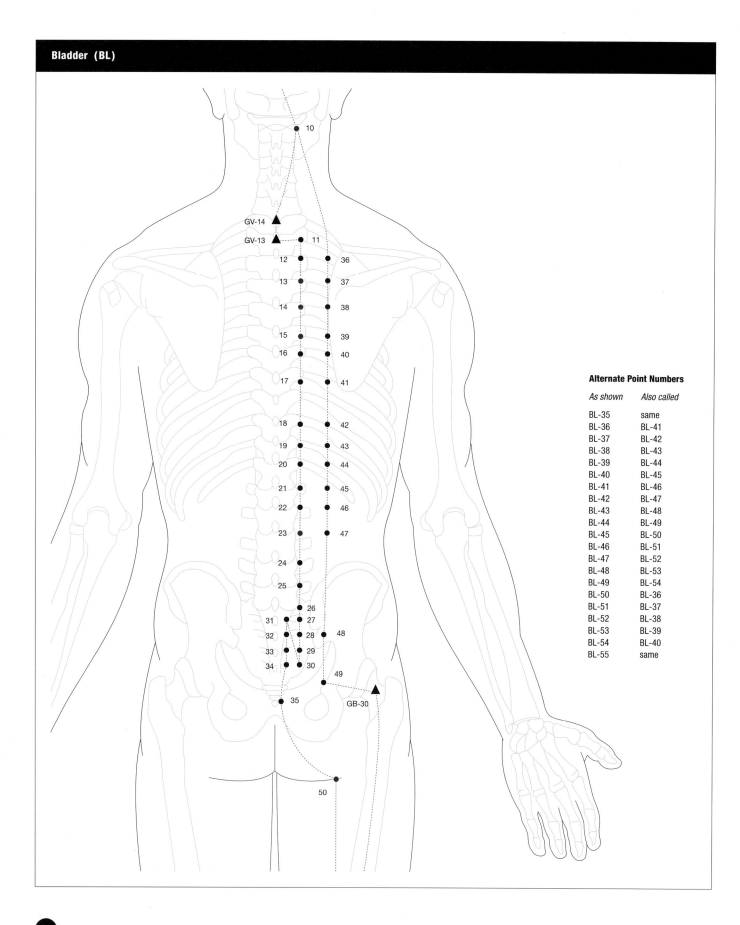

Alternate Point Numbers

As shown	Also called
BL-35	same
BL-36	BL-41
BL-37	BL-42
BL-38	BL-43
BL-39	BL-44
BL-40	BL-45
BL-41	BL-46
BL-42	BL-47
BL-43	BL-48
BL-44	BL-49
BL-45	BL-50
BL-46	BL-51
BL-47	BL-52
BL-48	BL-53
BL-49	BL-54
BL-50	BL-36
BL-51	BL-37
BL-52	BL-38
BL-53	BL-39
BL-54	BL-40
BL-55	same

Symbol	Chinese Name	Korean Japanese	Location	Local Anatomy (Nerves and Blood Vessels)
BL-24	Qi Hai Shu - Sea-of-Qi Shu	Gi Hae Yu Ki Kai Yu	Lower back, 1.5 units lateral to lower edge of spinous process of 3rd lumbar vertebra.	Lateral cutaneous branch of posterior ramus of 2nd lumbar nerve, posterior rami of 3rd lumbar artery and vein.
BL-25	Da Chang Shu - Large Intestine Shu	Dae Jang Yu Dai Cho Yu	Lower back, 1.5 units lateral to lower edge of spinous process of 4th lumbar vertebra.	Posterior ramus of 3rd lumbar nerve, posterior rami of 4th lumbar artery and vein.
BL-26	Guan Yuan Shu - Origin Pass Shu	Gwan Weon Yu Kan Gen Yu	Lower back, 1.5 units lateral to lower edge of spinous process of 5th lumbar vertebra.	Posterior ramus of 5th lumbar nerve, posterior branches of lowest lumbar artery and vein.
BL-27	Xiao Chang Shu - Small Intestine Shu	So Jang Yu Sho Cho Yu	Lower back, 1.5 units lateral to body midline (GV), level with 1st sacral foramen.	Lateral branch of posterior ramus of 1st sacral nerve, posterior branches of lateral sacral artery and vein.
BL-28	Pang Guang Shu - Bladder Shu	Bang Gwang Yu Bo Ko Yu	Lower back, 1.5 units lateral to body midline (GV), level with 2nd sacral foramen.	Lateral branches of posterior rami of 1st and 2nd sacral nerves, posterior branches of lateral sacral artery and vein.
BL-29	Zhong Lu Shu - Central Backbone Shu	Jung Lyeo Yu Chu Ryo Nai Yu	Lower back, 1.5 units lateral to body midline (GV), level with 3rd sacral foramen.	Lateral branches of posterior rami of 3rd and 4th sacral nerves, posterior branches of lateral sacral artery and vein, branches of inferior gluteal artery and vein.
BL-30	Bai Huan Shu - White Ring Shu	Baeg Hwang Yu Haku Kan Yu	Lower back, 1.5 units lateral to body midline (GV), level with 4th sacral foramen.	Lateral branches of posterior rami of 3rd and 4th sacral nerves, inferior gluteal nerve, inferior gluteal artery and vein, internal pudendal artery and vein (deeper).
BL-31	Shang Liao - Upper Bone-Hole	Sang Ryo Jo Ryo	Lower back, in 1st sacral foramen, between upper edge of iliac spine and midline.	Place where posterior ramus of 1st sacral nerve passes, posterior branches of lateral sacral artery and vein.
BL-32	Ci Liao - Second Bone-Hole	Cha Ryo Ji Ryo	Lower back, in 2nd sacral foramen, between lower edge of iliac spine and midline.	Course of posterior ramus of 2nd sacral nerve, posterior branches of lateral sacral artery and vein.
BL-33	Zhong Liao - Central Bone-Hole	Jung Ryo Chu Ryo	Lower back, in 3rd sacral foramen, between BL-29 and body midline.	Course of posterior ramus of 3rd sacral nerve, posterior branches of lateral sacral artery and vein.
BL-34	Xia Liao - Lower Bone-Hole	Ha Ryo Ge Ryo	Lower back, in 4th sacral foramen, between BL-30 and body midline.	Course of posterior ramus of 4th sacral nerve, branches of inferior gluteal artery and vein.
BL-35	Hui Yang - Meeting of Yang	Hoe Yang E Yo	Lower back, 0.5 unit lateral to body midline, level with tip of coccyx (tailbone).	Coccygeal nerve, branches of inferior gluteal artery and vein.
BL-36 [41]	Fu Fen - Attached Branch	Bu Bun Fu Bun	Upper back, 3 units lateral to lower edge of spinous process of 2nd thoracic vertebra.	Lateral cutaneous branches of posterior rami of 1st + 2nd thoracic n., dorsal scapular nerve (deeper), branch of transverse cervical a., sub-branches of intercostal a. and v.
BL-37 [42]	Po Hu - Po Door	Baek Ho Hakko	Upper back, 3 units lateral to lower edge of spinous process of 3rd thoracic vertebra.	Medial cutaneous branches of posterior rami of 2nd + 3rd thoracic n., dorsal scapular n. (deeper), posterior branch of intercostal a. , dec. branch of transverse cervical a.
BL-38 [43]	Gao Huang Shu - Vital Shu	Go Hwang Yu Ko Ko Yu	Upper back, 3 units lateral to lower edge of spinous process of 4th thoracic vertebra.	Medial cutaneous branches of posterior rami of 3rd + 4th thoracic n., dorsal scapular n. (deeper), posterior branch of intercostal a. , dec. branch of transverse cervical a.
BL-39 [44]	Shen Tang - Spirit Hall	Sin Dang Shin Do	Upper back, 3 units lateral to lower edge of spinous process of 5th thoracic vertebra.	Medial cutaneous branches of posterior rami of 4th + 5th thoracic n., dorsal scapular n. (deeper), posterior branches of intercostal a. + v., branch of transverse cervical a.
BL-40 [45]	Yi Xi - Surprise	Eui Heui I Ki	Upper back, 3 units lateral to lower edge of spinous process of 6th thoracic vertebra.	Medial cutaneous branches of posterior rami of 5th + 6th thoracic nerves, their lateral branches (deeper), posterior branches of intercostal artery and vein.
BL-41 [46]	Ge Guan - Diaphragm Pass	Gyeog Gwan Kaku Kan	3 units lateral to lower edge of spinous process of 7th thoracic vertebra, level to scapula base.	Medial cutaneous branches of posterior rami of 6th + 7th thoracic nerves, their lateral branches (deeper), posterior branches of intercostal artery and vein.
BL-42 [47]	Hun Men - Soul Gate	Hon Mun Kom Mon	Back, 3 units lateral to lower edge of spinous process of 9th thoracic vertebra.	Lateral branches of posterior rami of 7th + 8th thoracic nerves, posterior branches of intercostal artery and vein.
BL-43 [48]	Yang Gang - Yang Headrope	Yang Gang Yo Ko	Back, 3 units lateral to lower edge of spinous process of 10th thoracic vertebra.	Lateral branches of posterior rami of 8th + 9th thoracic nerves, posterior branches of intercostal artery and vein.
BL-44 [49]	Yi She - Reflection Abode	Eui Sa I Sha	Back, 3 units lateral to lower edge of spinous process of 11th thoracic vertebra.	Lateral branches of posterior rami of 10th + 11th thoracic nerves, posterior branches of intercostal artery and vein.
BL-45 [50]	Wei Cang - Stomach Granary	Wi Chang I So	Back, 3 units lateral to lower edge of spinous process of 12th thoracic vertebra.	Lateral branch of posterior ramus of 11th thoracic nerve, posterior branches of subcostal artery and vein.
BL-46 [51]	Huang Men - Vital Gate	Whang Mun Ko Mon	Back, 3 units lateral to lower edge of spinous process of 1st lumbar vertebra.	Lateral branch of 12th thoracic nerve, posterior branches of 1st lumbar artery and vein.

Small Numbers: Designate alternate acupoint numbers sometimes used to describe the same point.

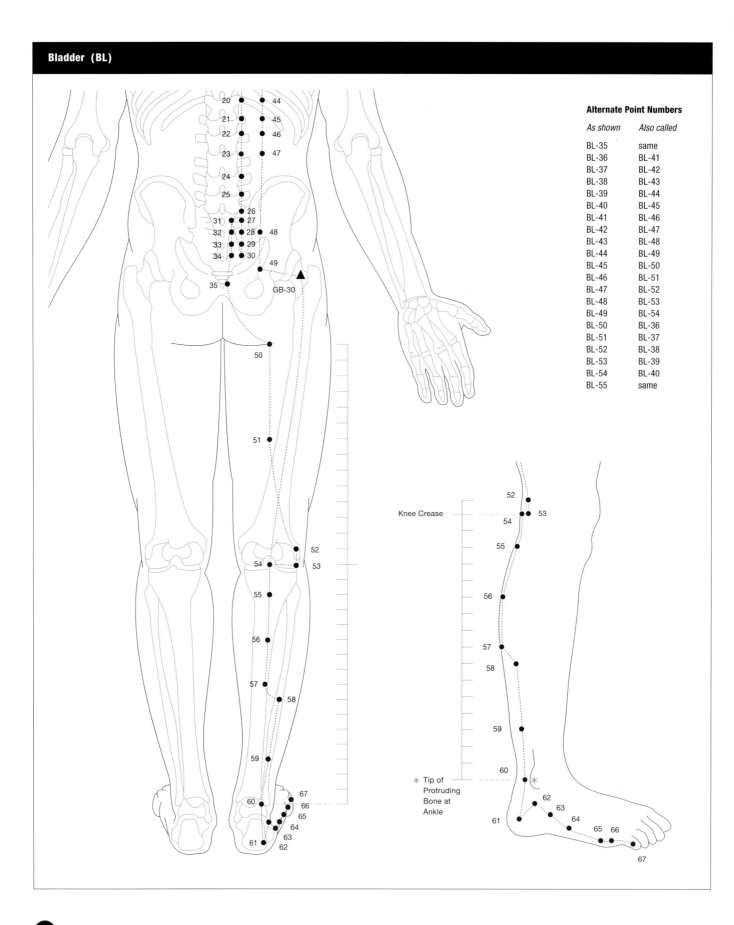

Alternate Point Numbers

As shown	Also called
BL-35	same
BL-36	BL-41
BL-37	BL-42
BL-38	BL-43
BL-39	BL-44
BL-40	BL-45
BL-41	BL-46
BL-42	BL-47
BL-43	BL-48
BL-44	BL-49
BL-45	BL-50
BL-46	BL-51
BL-47	BL-52
BL-48	BL-53
BL-49	BL-54
BL-50	BL-36
BL-51	BL-37
BL-52	BL-38
BL-53	BL-39
BL-54	BL-40
BL-55	same

Knee Crease

* Tip of Protruding Bone at Ankle

Bladder (BL)

Symbol	Chinese Name	Korean Japanese	Location	Local Anatomy (Nerves and Blood Vessels)
BL-47 52	Zhi Shi - Will Chamber	Ji Sil Shi Shitsu	Back, 3 units lateral to lower edge of spinous process of 2nd lumbar vertebra.	Lateral branch of posterior ramus of 12th thoracic nerve, lateral branch of 1st lumbar nerve.
BL-48 53	Bao Huang - Bladder Huang	Po Whang Ho Ko	Back, 3 units lateral to body midline, level with 2nd sacral foramen and BL-32.	Superior cluneal nerves, superior gluteal nerve (deeper), superior gluteal artery and vein.
BL-49 54	Zhi Bian - Sequential Limit	Jil Byeon Chippen	Lower back, 3 units lateral to body midline and sacral hiatus, directly below BL-48.	Inferior gluteal nerve, posterior femoral cutaneous nerve, sciatic nerve, inferior gluteal artery and vein.
• BL-50 36	Cheng Fu - Support	Seung Bu Sho Fu	Buttock, at midpoint of crease below buttock (transverse gluteal crease).	Posterior femoral cutaneous nerve (near surface), sciatic nerve (deeper), artery and vein running next to the sciatic nerve.
• BL-51 37	Yin Men - Gate of Abundance	Eun Mun Im Mon	Back of thigh, 6 units below BL-50 on line joining BL-50 to BL-54.	Posterior femoral cutaneous nerve, 3rd perforating branches of deep femoral artery and vein (slightly lateral).
BL-52 38	Fu Xi - Superficial Cleft	Bu Geug Fu Geki	Back of thigh, 1 unit above BL-53, at medial side of biceps femoris tendon (knee flexed).	Posterior femoral cutaneous nerve, common peroneal nerve, superolateral genicular artery and vein.
BL-53 39	Wei Yang - Bend Yang	Wi Yang I Yo	Back of knee, on the popliteal crease, at medial edge of biceps femoris tendon (knee flexed).	See BL-52.
• BL-54 40	Wei Zhong - Bend Middle	Wi Jung I Chu	Back of knee, midpoint of transverse crease, between biceps + semitendinosus m. tendons.	Posterior femoral cutaneous nerve, tibial nerve, femoropopliteal vein (near surface) popliteal vein (deeper and medial), popliteal artery (very deep).
BL-55	He Yang - Yang Union	Hab Yang Go Yo	Lower leg, 2 units directly below BL-54, between medial and lateral heads of gastrocnemius m.	Medial sural cutaneous nerve, tibial nerve (deeper), small saphenous vein, popliteal artery and vein (deeper).
• BL-56	Cheng Jin - Sinew Support	Seung Geun Sho Kin	Lower leg, halfway between BL-55 and BL-57, in center of belly of gastrocnemius m. (calf).	Medial sural cutaneous nerve, tibial nerve (deeper), small saphenous vein, posterior tibial artery and vein (deeper).
• BL-57	Cheng Shan - Mountain Support	Seung San Sho Zan	Lower leg, directly below belly of gastrocnemius muscle, on line joining BL-54 to Achilles tendon.	See BL-56.
BL-58	Fei Yang - Taking Flight	Bi Yang Hi Yo	Lower leg, at posterior edge of fibula bone, 1 unit lateral + down from BL-57, 7 units above BL-60.	Lateral sural cutaneous nerve.
BL-59	Fu Yang - Instep Yang	Bu Yang Fu Yo	Lower leg, 3 units directly above BL-60, at lateral side of gastrocnemius muscle.*	Sural nerve, small saphenous vein, terminal branch of peroneal artery (deeper). *Note: BL-59 is located on line joining BL-58 to BL-60.
• BL-60	Kun Lun - Kunlun Mountains	Gon Lyun Kon Ron	Outer ankle, recess halfway between protruding bone at ankle and Achilles tendon, level with tip.	Sural nerve, small saphenous vein, posteroexternal malleolar artery and vein (light pulse is felt).
BL-61	Pu Can - Subservient Visitor	Bog Sam Boku Shin	Outer heel, below BL-60 in recess at heel bone (calcaneus), at edge of red and white skin.	External calcaneal branch of sural nerve, external calcaneal branch of peroneal artery and vein.
BL-62	Shen Mai - Extending Vessel	Sin Maeg Shim Myaku	Outer foot, in recess directly below protruding bone at ankle (external malleolus).	Sural nerve, external malleolar arterial network.
BL-63	Jin Men - Metal Gate	Geum Mun Kim Mon	Outer foot, in recess below cuboid bone, forward and down (anterior and inferior) from BL-62.	Lateral dorsal cutaneous nerve of foot, lateral plantar nerve (deeper), lateral plantar artery and vein.
BL-64	Jing Gu - Capital Bone	Gyeong Gol Kei Kotsu	Outer side of foot, in recess below large bone, proximal to tuberosity of 5th metatarsal bone.	See BL-63.
BL-65	Shu Gu - Bundle Bone	Sog Gol Sokkotsu	Outer side of small toe, in recess behind base joint (proximal to head of 5th metatarsal bone).	4th common plantar digital nerve, lateral dorsal cutaneous nerve of foot, 4th common plantar digital artery and vein.
BL-66	Tong Gu - Valley Passage	Tong Gog Tsu Koku	Outer side of small toe, in recess in front of base joint (distal to 5th metatarsophalangeal joint).	Plantar digital proprial nerve, lateral dorsal cutaneous nerve of foot, plantar digital artery and vein.
BL-67	Zhi Yin - Reaching Yin	Ji Eum Shi In	Outer side of small toe, about 0.1 unit proximal to corner of nail.	Plantar digital proprial nerve, lateral dorsal cutaneous nerve of foot, network formed by dorsal digital artery and plantar digital proprial artery.

Small Numbers: Designate alternate acupoint numbers sometimes used to describe the same point.

Kidney (KI)

Primary Paths

The Kidney meridian begins beneath the little toe, crosses the sole of the foot, emerges at the arch (KI-2), circles behind the inner ankle, and passes through the heel. It then ascends the inner leg, intersecting SP-6, as it rises to the base of the spine to intersect GV-1. Here it ascends internally to enter its home Organ, the Kidney, after which it descends to connect with the Bladder and intersect CO-4 and CO-3. It returns to the surface above the pubic bone and ascends the front of the trunk, ending just below the clavicle head at the sternum (KI-27). An internal branch ascends from the Kidney, runs through the Liver and diaphragm, enters the Lung, and follows the throat to the root of the tongue. A short branch separates in the Lung, joins the Heart and disperses Qi in the chest.

Function

Kidney acupoints influence the ears, throat, waist, urogenital system, bone, head hair, general mental states, and the body's management of fluids.

Key Data

Type:	Yin
Phase:	Water
Acupoints:	27 (x2)
Qi-Flow:	5 pm – 7 pm
Connects with:	Bladder
Communication:	Heart

Special Points

Source-Yuan:	KI-3
Connecting-Luo:	KI-4
Cleft-Xi:	KI-5
Alarm-Mu:	GB-25
Associated-Shu:	BL-23

Intersection-Jiaohui Points

Penetrating ---	KI-11 to 21
Yin Linking ---	KI-9
Yin Heel ---	KI-6, 8

Points intersecting Kidney:
CO-3, 4, 17
GV-1
SP-6

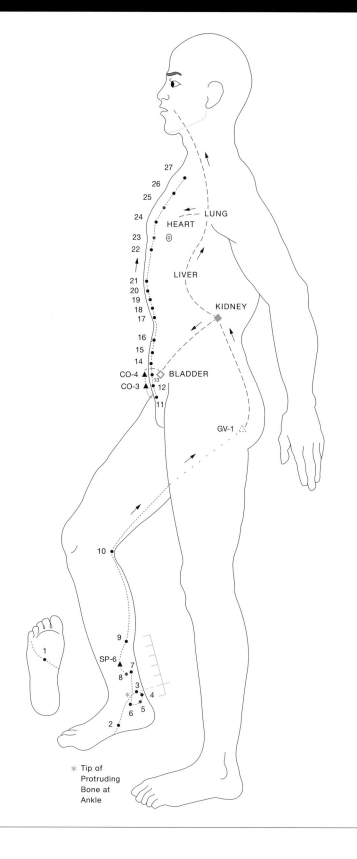

✳ Tip of Protruding Bone at Ankle

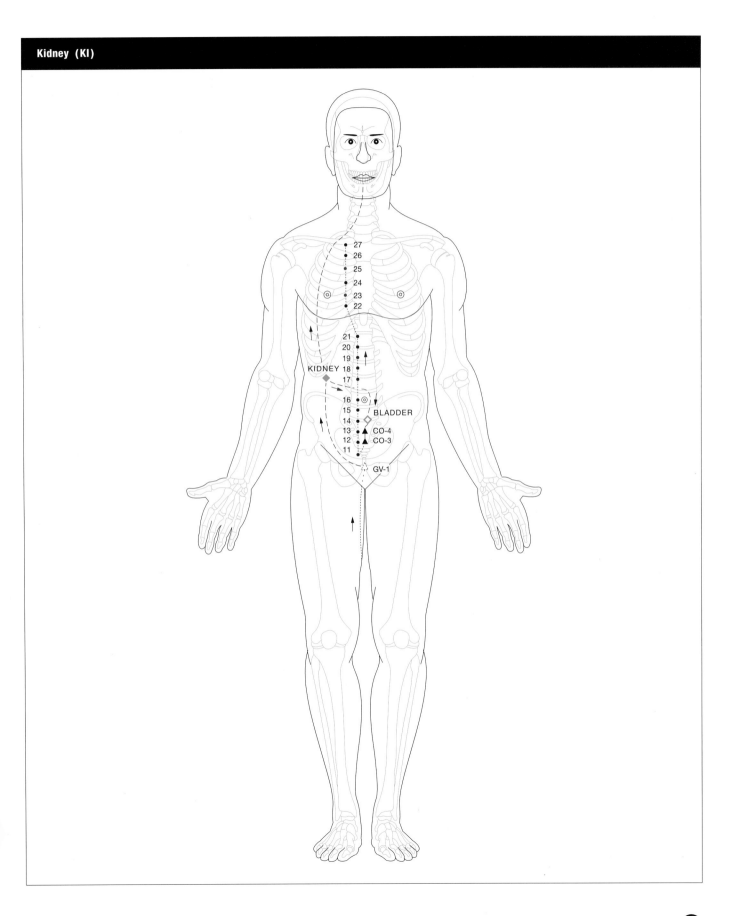

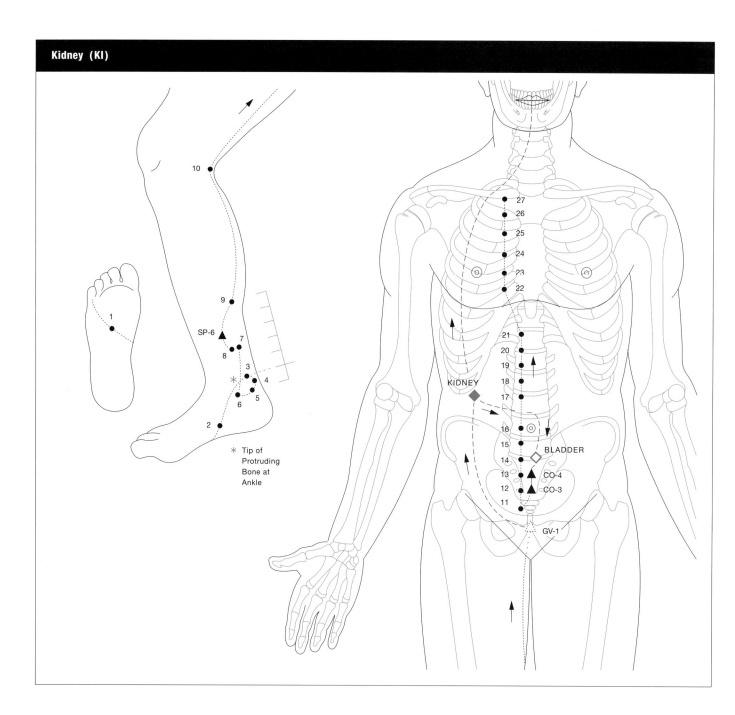

Symbol	Chinese Name	Korean Japanese	Location	Local Anatomy (Nerves and Blood Vessels)
KI-1	Yong Quan - Gushing Spring	Yong Cheon Yu Sen	Sole of foot, in recess 1/3 the distance from base of toes to heel, find with foot bent + toes curled.	2nd common plantar digital nerve, plantar arch (deeper).
KI-2	Ran Gu - Blazing Valley	Yeon Gog Nen Koku	Inner side of foot, in recess below lower edge of large bone (navicular) in front of inner ankle.	Terminal branch of medial crural cutaneous nerve, medial plantar nerve, branches of medial plantar and medial tarsal arteries.
KI-3	Tai Xi - Great Ravine	Tae Gye Tai Kei	Inner ankle, in recess between protruding bone at ankle and Achilles tendon, level with tip.	Medial crural cutaneous nerve, on course of tibial nerve, posterior tibial artery and vein (slightly anterior), pulse is felt.
KI-4	Da Zhong - Large Goblet	Dae Jong Tai Sho	0.5 unit below + slightly behind KI-3, between medial edge of Achilles tendon and heel bone.	Medial crural cutaneous nerve, on course of medial calcaneal ramus derived from tibial nerve, medial calcaneal branch of posterior tibial artery.

Kidney (KI)

Symbol	Chinese Name	Korean Japanese	Location	Local Anatomy (Nerves and Blood Vessels)
• KI-5	Shui Quan - Water Spring	Su Cheon Sui Sen	Inner heel, in recess above and in front of bulge in heel bone, 1 unit directly below KI-3.	See KI-4.
KI-6	Zhao Hai - Shining Sea	Jo Hae Sho Kai	Inner side of foot, in recess 1 unit below tip of protruding bone at ankle (medial malleolus).	Medial crural cutaneous nerve, tibial nerve (deeper), posterior tibial artery and vein (slightly posterior and inferior).
KI-7	Fu Liu - Recover Flow	Bu Lyu Fuku Ryu	Inner lower leg, in recess on front (anterior) edge of Achilles tendon, 2 units above KI-3.	Medial sural and medial crural cutaneous nerves, tibial nerve (deeper), posterior tibial artery and vein (deep and slightly anterior).
• KI-8	Jiao Xin - Intersection Reach	Gyo Sin Ko Shin	Inner lower leg, 2 units above KI-3, 0.5 unit anterior to KI-7, posterior to medial edge of tibia.	Medial crural cutaneous nerves, tibial nerve (deeper), posterior tibial artery and vein (deeper).
KI-9	Zhu Bin - Guest House	Chug Bin Chiku Hin	Inner lower leg, at lower inner edge of body of gastrocnemius m. (calf), 5 units above KI-3.	Medial sural cutaneous nerve, and medial crural cutaneous nerve, tibial nerve (deeper), posterior tibial artery and vein (deeper).
KI-10	Yin Gu - Yin Valey	Eum Gog In Koku	Medial side of back of knee, between semitendinosus + semimembranosus tendons, level BL-54.	Medial femoral cutaneous nerve, medial superior genicular artery and vein.
KI-11	Heng Gu - Pubic Bone	Hoeng Gol O Kotsu	In moon-shaped recess 5 units below navel, at upper edge of pubic bone, 0.5 unit lateral CO-2.	Branch of iliohypogastric nerve, inferior epigastric artery and external pudendal artery.
KI-12	Da He - Great Manifestation	Dae Hyeog Tai Kaku	Abdomen, 4 units below navel, 0.5 unit lateral CO-3.	Branches of subcostal nerve and iliohypogastric nerve, muscular branches of inferior epigastric artery and vein.
KI-13	Qi Xue - Qi Hole	Gi Hyeol Ki Ketsu	Abdomen, 3 units below navel, 0.5 unit lateral CO-4.	See KI-12.
KI-14	Si Man - Fourfold Fullness	Sa Man Shi Man	Abdomen, 2 units below navel, 0.5 unit lateral CO-5.	See KI-12.
KI-15	Zhong Zhu - Central Flow	Jung Ju Chu Chu	Abdomen, 1 unit below navel, 0.5 unit lateral CO-7.	10th intercostal nerve, muscular branches of inferior epigastric artery and vein.
KI-16	Huang Shu - Vital Shu	Hwang Yu Ko Yu	Abdomen, 0.5 unit lateral to center of navel (CO-8).	10th intercostal nerve, muscular branches of inferior epigastric artery and vein.
KI-17	Shang Qu - Shang Bend	Seog Gwan Sho Kyoku	Abdomen, 2 units above navel, 0.5 unit lateral CO-10.	9th intercostal nerve, branches of superior and inferior epigastric artery and vein.
KI-18	Shi Guan - Stone Pass	Sang Gog Seki Kan	Abdomen, 3 units above navel, 0.5 unit lateral CO-11.	8th intercostal nerve, branches of superior epigastric artery and vein.
KI-19	Yin Du - Yin Metropolis	Eum Do In To	Abdomen, 4 units above navel, 0.5 unit lateral CO-12.	See KI-18.
KI-20	Tong Gu - Open Valley	Tong Gog (Bok) Tsu Koku	Abdomen, 5 units above navel, 0.5 unit lateral CO-13.	See KI-18.
KI-21	You Men - Dark Gate	Yu Mun Yu Mon	Abdomen, 6 units above navel, 0.5 unit lateral CO-14.	7th intercostal nerve, branches of superior epigastric artery and vein.
KI-22	Bu Lang - Corridor Walk	Bo Rang Ho Ro	Chest, in 5th intercostal space (between ribs), 2 units lateral to Conception meridian (midline).	Anterior cutaneous branch of 5th intercostal nerve, 5th intercostal nerve (deeper), 5th intercostal artery and vein.
• KI-23	Shen Feng - Spirit Seal	Sin Bong Shim Po	Chest, in 4th intercostal space (between ribs), 2 units lateral to Conception meridian (midline).	Anterior cutaneous branch of 4th intercostal nerve, 4th intercostal nerve (deeper), 4th intercostal artery and vein, left bilateral acupoint is directly over heart.
KI-24	Ling Xu - Spirit Ruins	Yeong Heo Rei Kyo	Chest, in 3rd intercostal space (between ribs), 2 units lateral to Conception meridian (midline).	Anterior cutaneous branch of 3rd intercostal nerve, 3rd intercostal nerve (deeper), 3rd intercostal artery and vein.
• KI-25	Shen Cang - Spirit Storehouse	Sin Jang Shin Zo	Chest, in 2nd intercostal space (between ribs), 2 units lateral to Conception meridian (midline).	Anterior cutaneous branch of 2nd intercostal nerve, 2nd intercostal nerve (deeper), 2nd intercostal artery and vein.
KI-26	Yu Zhong - Lively Center	Ug Jung Waku Chu	Chest, in 1st intercostal space (between ribs), 2 units lateral to Conception meridian (midline).	Anterior cutaneous branch of 1st intercostal nerve, medial supraclavicular nerve, 1st intercostal nerve (deeper), 1st intercostal artery and vein.
KI-27	Shu Fu - Shu Mansion	Yu Bu Yu Fu	Chest, in recess at lower edge of medial head of clavicle, 2 units lateral to Conception meridian.	Medial supraclavicular nerve, anterior perforating branches of internal mammary artery and vein.

Pericardium (PC)

Primary Paths

The Pericardium meridian begins in the chest, where it enters its home Organ, the Pericardium. It descends internally through the diaphragm and into the abdominal cavity, sequentially connecting to the Upper, Middle and Lower Burners of the Triple Warmer. Another internal branch travels laterally from the Pericardium, across the chest, and emerges to the surface near the nipple (PC-1). From here, the external pathway ascends to the armpit, turns downward, and descends along the middle of the inner arm to the palm of the hand, ending at the radial side of the middle fingertip (PC-9). A short branch separates at the palm and runs to the end of the fourth finger (ring finger), where it connects with the Triple Warmer meridian. Some healing arts use alternate English names for the Pericardium meridian, such as *Heart Protector, Heart Constrictor* and *Circulation/Sex.*

Function

Pericardium acupoints influence the chest, heart, stomach and general mental states, and relate to fever diseases.

Key Data

Type:	Yin
Phase:	Fire
Acupoints:	9 (x2)
Qi-Flow:	7 pm – 9 pm
Connects with:	Triple Warmer
Communication:	Liver

Special Points

Source-Yuan:	PC-7
Connecting-Luo:	PC-6
Cleft-Xi:	PC-4
Alarm-Mu:	CO-17
Associated-Shu:	BL-14

Intersection-Jiaohui Points

Gallbladder —	PC-1

Points intersecting Pericardium:
CO-3, 4

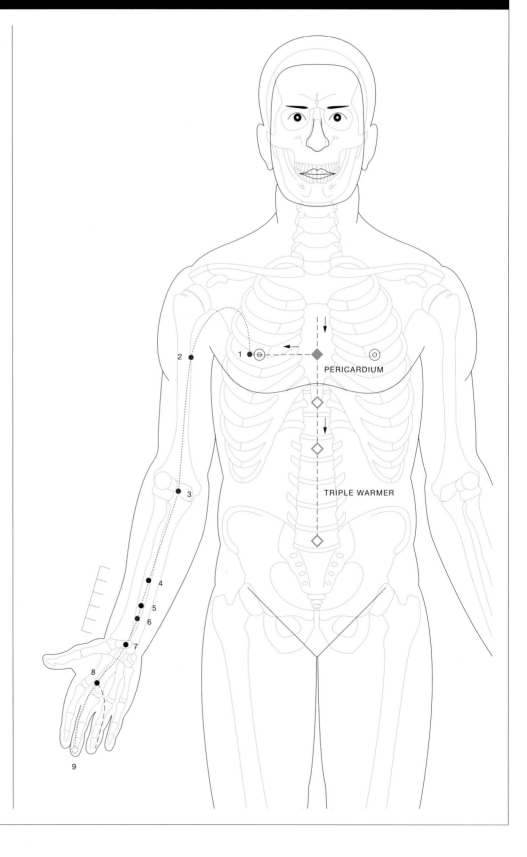

Pericardium (PC)

Symbol	Chinese Name	Korean Japanese	Location	Local Anatomy (Nerves and Blood Vessels)
• PC-1	Tian Chi - Celestial Pool	Cheon Ji Ten Chi	Chest, 1 unit lateral to nipple, in 4th intercostal space.	Muscular branch of anterior thoracic nerve, 4th intercostal nerve, thoracoepigastric vein, branches of lateral thoracic artery and vein.
• PC-2	Tian Quan - Celestial Spring	Cheon Cheon Ten Sen	Upper arm, 2 units below axillary (armpit) fold, between two heads of biceps brachii muscle.	Medial brachial cutaneous nerve, musculocutaneous nerve, muscular branches of brachial artery and vein.
• PC-3	Qu Ze - Marsh at the Bend	Gog Taeg Kyoku Taku	Inner elbow, on transverse crease, slightly medial to tendon of biceps brachii muscle.	Median nerve, path of brachial artery and vein.
PC-4	Xi Men - Cleft Gate	Geug Mun Geki Mon	5 units above wrist crease, between long palmar + radial flexor tendons, on line joining PC-3 to 7.	Medial antebrachial cutaneous nerve, median nerve (deeper), anterior interosseous nerve (very deep), median artery and vein, anterior interosseous a. and v. (deeper).
PC-5	Jian Shi - Intermediary Courier	Gan Sa Kan Shi	Forearm, 3 units above wrist crease, between tendons of long palmar m. and radial flexor m.	Medial+lateral antebrachial cutaneous n., palmar cut. branch of median n., anterior interosseous n. (very deep), median a. and v., anterior interosseous a. and v. (deep).
• PC-6	Nei Guan - Inner Pass	Nae Gwan Nai Kan	Forearm, 2 units above wrist crease, between tendons of long palmar m. and radial flexor m.	See PC-5.
PC-7	Da Ling - Great Mound	Dae Leung Tai Ryo	Wrist, in recess at middle of wrist crease, between tendons (long palmar+radial flexor).	Median nerve (deeper), palmar arterial and venous network of wrist.
PC-8	Lao Gong - Palace of Toil	No Gung Ro Kyu	Palm, between 2nd and 3rd metacarpal bones, at radial side of 3rd, proximal to base joint of finger.	2nd common palmar digital nerve of median nerve, common palmar digital artery.
PC-9	Zhong Chong - Central Hub	Jung Chung Chu Sho	Radial side of middle finger, about 0.1 unit above (proximal) corner of nail.	Palmar digital proprial nerve of median nerve, arterial and venous network formed by palmar digital proprial artery and vein.

Triple Warmer (TW)

Primary Paths

The Triple Warmer meridian begins externally, at the tip of the fourth finger (TW-1). It ascends the outer arm to the shoulder and upper back, sequentially intersecting SI-12, GV-14 and GB-21. From here, it enters the body, passes through the chest and intersects CO-17. It then connects with the Pericardium and descends internally, entering the Upper, Middle and Lower Burners of the Triple Warmer (home Organ). A branch of the main meridian, separates at CO-17 and ascends internally, surfacing at the neck. It ascends behind the ear, intersects GB-6 and GB-4, and circles the face to end at SI-18. Another branch separates behind the ear lobe, enters the ear, emerges in front, and crosses to the eyebrow to end at TW-23.

Function

Triple Warmer acupoints influence the eyes, ears, throat, and water metabolism, and relate to fever diseases.

Key Data

Type:	Yang
Phase:	Fire
Acupoints:	23 (x2)
Qi-Flow:	9 pm – 11 pm
Connects with:	Pericardium
Communication:	Gallbladder

Special Points

Source-Yuan:	TW-4
Connecting-Luo:	TW-5
Cleft-Xi:	TW-7
Alarm-Mu:	CO-5
Associated-Shu:	BL-22
Lower Uniting:	BL-53

Intersection-Jiaohui Points

Large Intestine —	TW-20
Small Intestine —	TW-22
Gallbladder —	TW-17, 20, 22
Conception ---	ST-1
Yang Linking —	TW-15
Yang Heel —	TW-15

Points intersecting Triple Warmer:

BL-53	GV-14
CO-12, 17	SI-12, 18, 19
GB-1,3, 4, 6, 21	

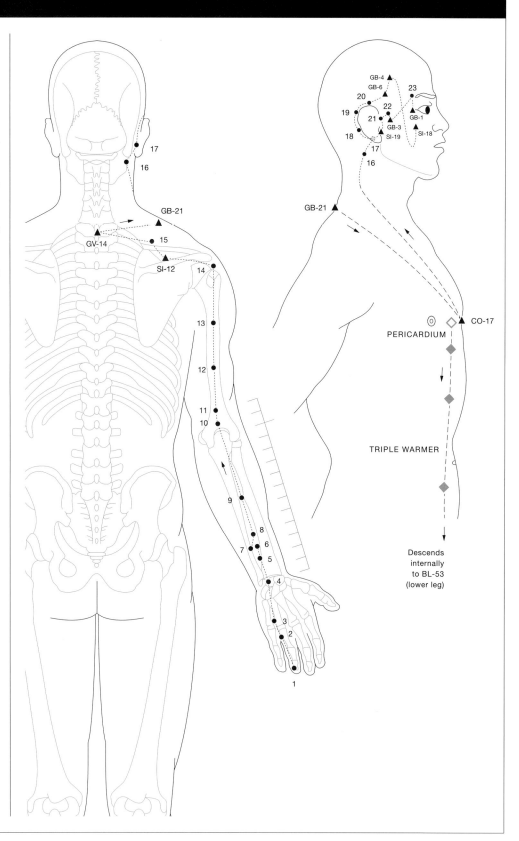

Triple Warmer (TW)

Symbol	Chinese Name	Korean Japanese	Location	Local Anatomy (Nerves and Blood Vessels)
TW-1	Guan Chong - Passage Hub	Gwan Chung Kan Sho	Ulnar side of ring finger, about 0.1 unit above (proximal) corner of nail.	Palmar digital proprial nerve from ulnar nerve, arterial and venous network formed by palmar digital proprial artery and vein.
TW-2	Ye Men - Humor Gate	Aeg Mun Eki Mon	Back of hand, between ring+small finger, above edge of web, near joint (locate on clenched fist).	Dorsal branch of ulnar nerve, dorsal digital artery of ulnar artery.
• TW-3	Zhong Zhu - Central Islet	Jung Jeo Chu Cho	Back of hand, between 4th and 5th metacarpal bones, in recess proximal base joints of fingers.	Dorsal branch of ulnar nerve, dorsal venous network of hand and 4th dorsal metacarpal artery.
TW-4	Yang Chi - Yang Pool	Yang Ji Yo Chi	Back of wrist, at junction of ulna + carpal bones, in recess lateral to extensor digitorum tendon.	Dorsal branch of ulnar nerve, terminal branch of posterior antebrachial cutaneous nerve, dorsal venous network of wrist and posterior carpal artery (slightly below).
• TW-5	Wai Guan - Outer Pass	Oe Gwan Gai Kan	Back of forearm, 2 units above TW-4, between radius and ulna bones, opposite PC-6.	Posterior antebrachial cutaneous n., posterior interosseous n. of radial n. and anterior interosseous n. of median n. (deeper), posterior + anterior interosseous a. and v.
TW-6	Zhi Gou - Branch Ditch	Ji Gu Shi Ko	Back of forearm, 3 units above TW-4, between radius and ulna bones.	See TW-5.
TW-7	Hui Zong - Meeting of the Clan	Hoe Jong E So	Back of forearm, 3 units above wrist, 0.75 unit lateral to TW-6, on radial side of ulna bone.	Posterior and medial antebrachial cutaneous nerves, posterior and anterior interosseous nerves (deeper), posterior interosseous artery and vein.
TW-8	San Yang Luo - Three Yang Connection	Sam Yang Rag San Yo Raku	Back of forearm, 4 units above TW-4, between radius and ulna bones.	See TW-7.
TW-9	Si Du - Four Rivers	Sa Dok Shi Toku	Back of forearm, 5 units below point of elbow (olecranon), between radius and ulna bones.	See TW-7.
TW-10	Tian Jing - Celestial Well	Cheon Jeong Ten Sei	Back of elbow, in recess about 1 unit above point of elbow (superior to olecranon), with elbow bent.	Posterior brachial cutaneous nerve, muscular branch of radial nerve, arterial and venous network of elbow.
• TW-11	Qing Leng Yuan - Clear Cold Abyss	Cheong Raeng Yeon Sei Rei En	Back of upper arm, 1 unit above TW-10.	Posterior brachial cutaneous nerve, muscular branch of radial nerve, terminal branches of median collateral artery and vein.
• TW-12	Xiao Luo - Dispersing Riverbed	So Rag Sho Reki	On line joining elbow point to TW-14, halfway between 11+13, at end of lateral head of triceps.	Posterior brachial cutaneous nerve, muscular branch of radial nerve, median collateral artery and vein.
TW-13	Nao Hui - Upper Arm Convergence	No Hoe Ju E	Upper arm at posterior edge of deltoid m., 3 units below TW-14, on line from elbow point to TW-14.	Posterior brachial cutaneous nerve, muscular branch of radial nerve, radial nerve (deeper), medial collateral artery and vein.
TW-14	Jian Liao - Shoulder Bone-Hole	Gyeon Ryo Ken Ryo	Back of shoulder, posterior and below protruding bone (acromion), in recess 1 unit behind LI-15.	Muscular branch of axillary nerve, muscular branch of posterior circumflex humeral artery.
• TW-15	Tian Liao - Celestial Bone-Hole	Cheon Ryo Ten Ryo	Above shoulder blade (scapula), halfway between GB-21 and SI-13.	Accessory nerve, branch of suprascapular nerve, descending branch of transverse cervical artery, muscular branch of suprascapular artery (deeper).
TW-16	Tian You - Celestial Oriole	Cheon Yu Ten Yo	Neck, below mastoid process, on rear edge of sternoceidomastoid m., level to SI-17 and BL-10.	Lesser occipital nerve, posterior auricular artery.
• TW-17	Yi Feng - Wind Screen	Ye Pung Ei Fu	In recess behind ear lobe, between mastoid process (on skull) and jawbone (mandible).	Great auricular nerve, place where facial nerves emerge from stylomastoid foramen (deeper), posterior auricular artery and vein, external jugular vein.
TW-18	Chi Mai - Spasm Vessel	Gye Maeg Kei Myaku	Behind base of ear, in center of mastoid process, 1/3 the distance on curve joining TW-17+TW-20.	Posterior auricular branch of great auricular nerve, posterior auricular artery and vein.
TW-19	Lu Xi - Skull Rest	No Sig Ro Soku	Behind ear, 2/3 the distance on curve joining TW-17 and TW-20.	Anastomotic branch of great auricular nerve, and lesser occipital nerve, posterior auricular artery and vein.
TW-20	Jiao Sun - Angle Vertex	Gag Son Kaku Son	Side of head, directly above apex of ear, within hairline (recess appears when mouth is open).	Branches of auriculotemporal nerve, branches of superficial temporal artery and vein.
TW-21	Er Men - Ear Gate	I Mun Ji Mon	Side of head, in recess anterior to upper notch of protruding flesh (tragus) in front of ear.	Branches of auriculotemporal and facial nerves, superficial temporal artery and vein.
TW-22	He Liao - Harmony Bone-Hole	Hwa Ryo Wa Ryo	Side of head, in front and above TW-21, level with root of ear, where a horizontal pulse is felt.	Branch of auriculotemporal nerve on course of temporal branch of facial nerve, superficial temporal artery and vein.
• TW-23	Si Zhu Kong - Silk Bamboo Hole	Sa Jug Gong Shi Chiku Ku	Side of head, in recess at lateral end of eyebrow.	Zygomatic branch of facial nerve, branch of auriculotemporal nerve, frontal branches of superficial temporal artery and vein.

Gallbladder (GB)

Primary Paths

The Gallbladder meridian begins at the outer corner of the eye (GB-1), where two branches originate: internal and external. The external branch follows a zig-zag circular path, back and forth across the head, intersecting points on the Triple Warmer and Stomach meridians, before descending below the ear to intersect SI-17. From here, it descends to the back of the shoulder, intersecting GV-14 and SI-12, before crossing over to ST-12 at the clavicle. From here, it descends externally to the hip, intersects BL-31 and BL-34, and runs down the outer leg, ending at the lateral tip of the fourth toe (GB-44). A short branch separates below the ankle (GB-41) and runs to the big toe, to connect with the Liver meridian. A short branch separates from the main path behind the ear, intersecting TW-17, SI-19 and ST-7, before ending at the outer corner of the eye.

The internal branch (starting at GB-1) circles the cheek, intersecting ST-5, before descending to ST-12 at the clavicle, where it meets the external branch. The internal branch descends through the chest, intersects PC-1, connects with the Liver, and enters its home Organ, the Gallbladder. It then run down into the groin area and joins the external path in the hip at GB-30.

Function

Gallbladder acupoints influence the eyes, ears, nose, mouth, and mental states, and relate to fever diseases.

Key Data

Type:	Yang
Phase:	Wood
Acupoints:	44 (x2)
Qi-Flow:	11 pm – 1 am
Connects with:	Liver
Communication:	Triple Warmer

Special Points

Source-Yuan:	GB-40
Connecting-Luo:	GB-37
Cleft-Xi:	GB-36
Alarm-Mu:	GB-24

Associated-Shu:	BL-19
Lower Uniting:	GB-34
Meeting-Hui (Tendons):	GB-34
Meeting-Hui (Marrow):	GB-39

Intersection-Jiaohui Points

Stomach —	GB-3, 6
Spleen ---	GB-24
Small Intestine —	GB-1
Bladder —	GB-7, 8, 10, 11, 12, 15, 30
Triple Warmer —	GB-1, 3, 4, 6, 21
Girdling —	GB-26, 27, 28
Yang Linking —	GB-13 to 21, 35
Yang Heel —	GB-20, 29

Points intersecting Gallbladder:

BL-31, 34	SI-12, 17, 19
GV-1, 14	ST-5, 7, 8, 12
LV-13	TW-17, 20, 22
PC-1	

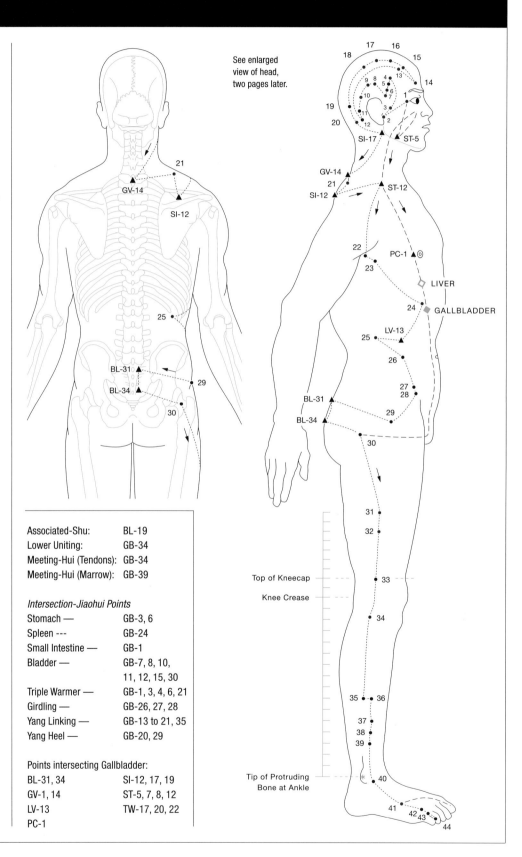

See enlarged view of head, two pages later.

Gallbladder (GB)

Symbol	Chinese Name	Korean Japanese	Location	Local Anatomy (Nerves and Blood Vessels)
• GB-1	Tong Zi Liao - Pupil Bone-Hole	Dong Ja Ryo Do Shi Ryo	About 0.5 unit lateral to outer corner of eye, in recess on lateral side of orbit (bony eye socket).	Zygomaticofacial and zygomaticotemporal nerves, temporal branch of facial nerve, zygomaticoorbital artery and vein.
• GB-2	Ting Hui - Auditory Convergence	Cheong Hoe Cho E	In recess anterior to lower notch of protruding flesh (tragus) in front of ear, below SI-19 (pulse).	Great auricular nerve, facial nerve, superficial temporal artery.
• GB-3	Shang Guan - Upper Gate	Gaek Ju In Kyaku Shu Jin	In front of ear, on upper edge of zygomatic arch (bone), above ST-7, recess when mouth is open.	Zygomatic branch of facial nerve and zygomaticofacial nerve, zygomaticoorbital artery and vein.
• GB-4	Han Yan - Forehead Fullness	Ham Yeom Gan En	Side of head, within hairline of temporal region, 1/4 the distance between ST-8 and GB-7.	Just on temporal branch of auriculotemporal nerve, parietal branches of superficial temporal artery and vein.
GB-5	Xuan Lu - Suspended Skull	Hyeon Ro Ken Ro	Side of head, within hairline of temporal region, halfway on a line joining ST-8 and GB-7.	See GB-4.
• GB-6	Xuan Li - Suspended Tuft	Hyeon Ri Ken Ri	Side of head, within hairline of temporal region, halfway on a line joining GB-5 and GB-7.	See GB-4.
• GB-7	Qu Bin - Temporal Hairline Curve	Gog Bin Kyoku Bin	Within hairline of temple, above and in front of ear, level with and 0.75 unit anterior to TW-20.	See GB-4.
• GB-8	Shuai Gu - Valley Lead	Sol Gog Sokkoku	Side of head, above apex of ear, in recess 1.5 units within hairline (point is felt when biting).	Anastomotic branch of auriculotemporal nerve and great occipital nerve, parietal branches of superficial temporal artery and vein.
• GB-9	Tian Chong - Celestial Hub	Cheon Chung Ten Sho	Side of head, above and behind ear, 2 units within hairline, about 0.5 unit behind GB-8.	Branch of great occipital nerve, posterior auricular artery and vein.
• GB-10	Fu Bai - Floating White	Bu Baeg Fu Haku	Behind ear and above mastoid process, 1 unit below and posterior to GB-9.	See GB-9.
GB-11	Tou Qiao Yin - Head Portal Yin	Du Gyu Eum Atama Kyo In	Behind ear and at base of mastoid process, about 1 unit below GB-10.	Anastomotic branch of great and lesser occipital nerves, branches of posterior auricular artery and vein.
GB-12	Wan Gu - Completion Bone	Wan Gol Kan Kotsu	In recess at posterior edge of mastoid process, within hair, 0.7 unit below GB-11, level to GV-16.	Lesser occipital nerve, posterior auricular artery and vein.
• GB-13	Ben Shen - Root Spirit	Bon Sin Hon Jin	3 units lateral to GV-24, 0.5 unit within hairline of forehead, 2/3 the distance from GV-24 to ST-8.	Lateral branch of frontal nerve, frontal branches of superficial temporal artery and vein, lateral branches of frontal artery and vein.
• GB-14	Yang Bai - Yang White	Yang Baek Yo Haku	Forehead, 1 unit above midpoint of eyebrow, aligned with eye pupil.	Lateral branch of frontal nerve, lateral branches of frontal artery and vein.
• GB-15	Tou Lin Qi - Head Overlooking Tears	Im Eub Atama Rin Kyu	Forehead, directly above GB-14, 0.5 unit within hairline, halfway between GV-24 and ST-8.	Anastomotic branch of medial and lateral branches of frontal nerve, frontal artery and vein.
• GB-16	Mu Chuang - Eye Window	Mog Chang Moku So	Head, 1.5 units posterior to GB-15, on line joining GB-15 to GB-20.	Anastomotic branch of medial and lateral branches of frontal nerve, frontal branches of superficial temporal artery and vein.
• GB-17	Zheng Ying - Upright Construction	Jeong Yeong Sho Ei	Head, 1.5 units posterior to GB-16, on line joining GB-15 to GB-20.	Anastomotic branch of frontal and great occipital nerves, anastomotic plexus formed by parietal branches of superficial temporal artery and vein and occipital a. and v.
• GB-18	Cheng Ling - Spirit Support	Seung Lyeong Sho Rei	On head, 1.5 units posterior to GB-17, on line joining GB-15 to GB-20.	Branch of great auricular nerve, branches of occipital artery and vein.
GB-19	Nao Kong - Brain Hollow	Noe Gong No Ku	Back of head, directly above GB-20, level with GV-17, lateral side of protruding occipital bone.	See GB-18.
• GB-20	Feng Chi - Wind Pool	Pung Ji Fu Chi	Back of neck, below occipital bone, in recess between sternoceidomastoid m. and trapezius m.	Branch of lesser occipital nerve, branches of occipital artery and vein.
• GB-21	Jian Jing - Shoulder Well	Gyeon Jeong Ken Sei	Shoulder, halfway between C7 vertebra and protruding bone at top of shoulder (acromion).	Lateral branch of supraclavicular nerve, accessory nerve, transverse cervical artery and vein.
GB-22	Yuan Ye - Armpit Abyss	Yeon Aeg En Eki	Side of trunk, in recess 3 units below armpit (axilla), on midaxillary line, 5th intercostal space.	Lateral cutaneous branch of 5th intercostal nerve, branch of long thoracic nerve, thoracoeepigastric vein, lateral thoracic artery and vein, 5th intercostal a. and v.
GB-23	Zhe Jin - Sinew Seat	Cheob Geun Shu Kin	Side of trunk, 1 unit anterior to GB-22, almost level with nipple.	Lateral cutaneous branch of 5th intercostal nerve, lateral thoracic artery and vein, 5th intercostal artery and vein.

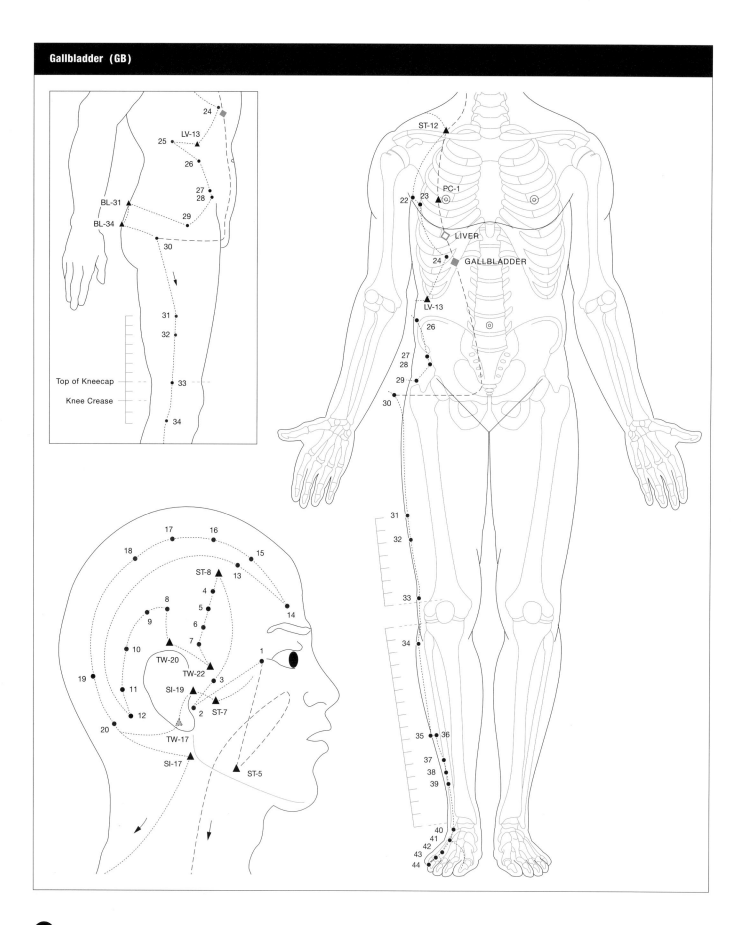

24

LV-13
25
26
27
28
29
BL-31
BL-34
30
31
32
Top of Kneecap
Knee Crease
33
34

ST-12
PC-1
22 23
LIVER
24 GALLBLADDER
LV-13
26
27
28
29
30
31
32
33
34
35 36
37
38
39
40
41
42
43
44

17 16
18   15
ST-8 13
4
8   5   14
9   6
7
10
TW-20
19   TW-22
11   SI-19   3   1
12   2   ST-7
20
TW-17
SI-17
ST-5

Gallbladder (GB)

Symbol	Chinese Name	Korean Japanese	Location	Local Anatomy (Nerves and Blood Vessels)
• GB-24	Ri Yue - Sun and Moon	Il Weol Jitsu Getsu	Below nipple, between cartilage of 7th+8th ribs, one rib space below and slightly lateral to LV-14.	7th intercostal nerve, 7th intercostal artery and vein.
• GB-25	Jing Men - Capital Gate	Gyeong Mun Kei Mon	Side of trunk, at lower edge of floating end of 12th rib (lowest rib).	11th intercostal nerve, 11th intercostal artery and vein.
GB-26	Dai Mai - Girdling Vessel	Dae Maeg Tai Myaku	Side of trunk, level with navel, vertically aligned with free end of 11th floating rib (LV-13).	Subcostal nerve, subcostal artery and vein.
GB-27	Wu Shu - Fifth Pivot	O Chu Go Su	Abdomen, on anterior side of front-upper iliac spine of hipbone, 3 units below level of navel.	Iliohypogastric nerve, superficial and deep circumflex iliac arteries and veins.
GB-28	Wei Dao - Linking Path	Yu Do Yui Do	0.5 unit below and slightly medial to GB-27, slightly below front-upper iliac spine of hipbone.	Ilioinguinal nerve, superficial and deep circumflex iliac arteries and veins.
GB-29	Ju Liao - Squating Bone-Hole	Geo Ryo Kyo Ryo	Halfway between front-upper iliac spine of hip-bone + protruding bone at upper leg (trochanter).	Lateral femoral cutaneous nerve, branches of superficial circumflex iliac artery and vein, ascending branches of lateral circumflex femoral artery and vein.
GB-30	Huan Tiao - Jumping Round	Hwan Jo Kan Cho	In hip joint, 1/3 the distance from greater trochanter to sacral hiatus (GV-2).	Inferior cluneal cutaneous nerve, inferior gluteal nerve, sciatic nerve (deeper), inferior gluteal artery and vein.
• GB-31	Feng Shi - Wind Market	Pung Si Fu Shi	Outer thigh, 7 units above kneecap, at end of middle finger when arm hangs at side.	Lateral femoral cutaneous nerve, muscular branch of femoral nerve, muscular branches of lateral circumflex femoral artery and vein.
• GB-32	Zhong Du - Central River	Jung Dog Chu Toku	Outer thigh, 2 units below GB-31, between vastus lateralis and biceps femoris muscles.	See GB-31.
GB-33	(Xi) Yang Guan - (Knee) Yang Joint	Yang Gwan (Oshi) Yo Kan	Outer thigh, in recess above bony knob of femur, between bone and biceps femoris tendon.*	Terminal branch of lateral femoral cutaneous nerve, superior lateral genicular artery and vein. *Note: GB-33 is located posterior to knee joint when knee is bent.
• GB-34	Yang Ling Quan - Yang Mound Spring	Yang Leung Cheon Yo Ryo Sen	Outer leg below knee, in recess anterior to and slightly below head of fibula bone (with leg bent).	Point where common peroneal nerve branches into superficial and deep peroneal nerves, inferior lateral genicular artery and vein.
GB-35	Yang Jiao - Yang Intersection	Yang Gyo Yo Ko	7 units above protruding bone tip at outer ankle, on rear edge of fibula, level with GB-36 + BL-58.	Lateral sural cutaneous nerve, branches of peroneal artery and vein.
GB-36	Wai Qiu - Outer Hill	Oe Gu Gai Kyu	7 units above protruding bone tip at outer ankle, on front edge of fibula, level with GB-35 + ST-39.	Superficial peroneal nerve, branches of anterior tibial artery and vein.
GB-37	Guang Ming - Bright Light	Gwang Myeong Ko Myo	5 units above protruding bone tip at outer ankle, on front edge of fibula, between muscles.*	See GB-36 *Note: Point is located between peroneus brevis + extensor digitorum longus muscles.
GB-38	Yang Fu - Yang Assistance	Yang Bo Yo Ho	4 units above + slightly in front of protruding bone tip at outer ankle, on front edge of fibula.	See GB-36.
GB-39	Xuan Zhong - Suspended Bell *	Hyeon Jong Ken Sho	3 units above tip of bone at outer ankle, in recess between peroneus tendons + rear edge of fibula.	See GB-36. *Note: In Chinese, this acupoint is also called *Jue Gu*, meaning "Severed Bone."
GB-40	Qiu Xu - Hill Ruins	Gu Heo Kyu Kyo	In recess, forward and below protruding bone at outer ankle, lateral side of long extensor tendon.	Branches of intermediate dorsal cutaneous nerve and superficial peroneal nerve, branch of antelateral malleolar artery.
• GB-41	(Zu) Lin Qi - (Foot) Overlooking Tears	(Jog) Im Eub (Ashi) Rin Kyu	Top of foot, in recess distal and between junction of 4th and 5th metatarsal bones.	Branch of intermediate dorsal cutaneous nerve of foot.
GB-42	Di Wu Hui - Earth Five-Fold	Ji O Hoe Chi Go E	Top of foot, between 4th+5th metatarsal bones, on medial side of extensor tendon of small toe.	See GB-41.
GB-43	Jia Xi - Pinched Ravine	Hyeob Gye Kyo Kei	Top of foot, distal and between base joints of 4th and 5th toes, in the web of little toe.	Dorsal digital nerve, dorsal digital artery and vein.
GB-44	(Zu) Qiao Yin - (Foot) Portal Yin	(Jog) Gyu Eum (Ashi) Kyo In	Lateral side of 4th toe, about 0.1 unit above (proximal) to corner of nail.	Dorsal digital nerve, arterial and venous network formed by dorsal digital artery and vein and plantar digital artery and vein.

Liver (LV)

Primary Paths

The Liver meridian begins externally, at the inside tip of the big toe (LV-1). It ascends in front of the inner ankle, intersects SP-6, and rises up the inner leg to the groin area, where it intersects SP-12 and SP-13. Then it encircles the genitals and intersects CO-2, CO-3 and CO-4. It continues up to the lower abdomen (LV-14), where it penetrates the body to enter its home Organ, the Liver, and connect with the Gallbladder. The internal path continues up across the diaphragm, ascends behind the throat, and connects with the tissue surrounding the eyes. It then ascends the forehead, ending at the vertex of the head, where it meets the Governing meridian. A short branch separates below the eye and circles the inner surface of the lips. Another branch splits off from the Liver and enters the Lung, to begin the entire Qi-flow cycle again.

Function

Liver acupoints influence the head, eyes, muscles, joints, tendons, nails, abdomen, endocrine functions, urogenital system, and mental states.

Key Data

Type: Yin
Phase: Wood
Acupoints: 14 (x2)
Qi-Flow: 1 am – 3 am
Connects with: Gallbladder
Communication: Pericardium

Special Points

Source-Yuan: LV-3
Connecting-Luo: LV-5
Cleft-Xi: LV-6
Alarm-Mu: LV-14
Associated-Shu: BL-18
Meeting-Hui
  (Yin Organs): LV-13

Intersection-Jiaohui Points

Spleen --- LV-14
Gallbladder — LV-13
Yin Linking --- LV-14

Points intersecting Liver:
CO-2, 3, 4   SP-6, 12, 13

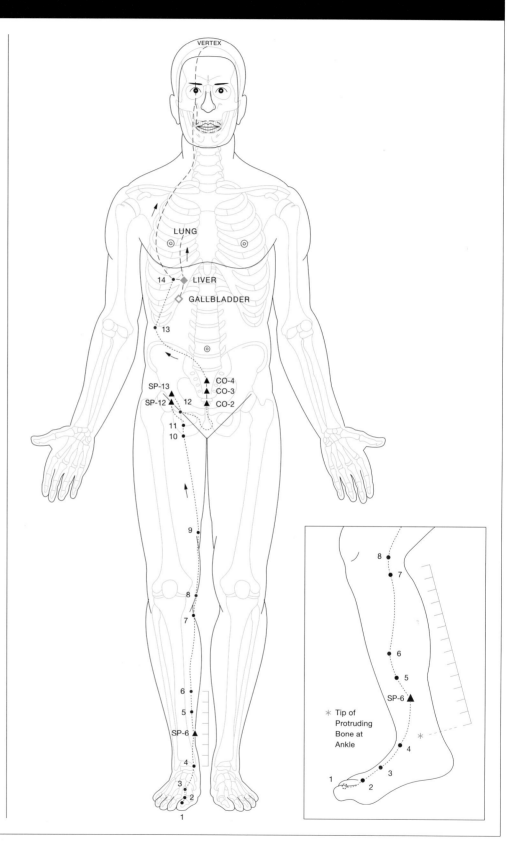

Liver (LV)

Symbol	Chinese Name	Korean Japanese	Location	Local Anatomy (Nerves and Blood Vessels)
LV-1	Da Dun - Large Pile	Tae Don Tai Ton	Lateral side of big toe, about 0.1 unit above (proximal) to corner of nail.	Dorsal digital nerve derived from deep peroneal nerve, dorsal digital artery and vein.
LV-2	Xing Jian - Moving Between	Haeng Gan Ko Kan	Top of foot, distal and between base joints of 1st and 2nd toe, in the web of big toe.	Place where dorsal digital nerves branch from deep peroneal nerve, dorsal venous network of foot, first digital artery and vein.
• LV-3	Tai Chong - Supreme Surge	Tae Chung Tai Sho	Top of foot, in recess distal and between junction of 1st and 2nd metatarsal bones (above web).	Branch of deep peroneal nerve, dorsal venous network of foot, first dorsal metatarsal artery.
LV-4	Zhong Feng - Mound Center	Jung Bong Chu Ho	1 unit anterior to lower edge of protruding bone at inner ankle, in recess between SP-5 + ST-41.	Branch of medial dorsal cutaneous nerve of foot and saphenous nerve, dorsal venous network of foot, anterior medial malleolar artery.
LV-5	Li Gou - Woodworm Canal	Yeo Gu Rei Ko	5 units above tip of protruding bone at inner ankle, between posterior edge of tibia and calf m.*	Branch of saphenous nerve, great saphenous vein (slightly posterior). *Note: LV-5 is located in a valley between tibia bone and gastrocnemius muscle.
• LV-6	Zhong Du - Central Metropolis	Jung Do Chu To	Inner ankle, 7 units above tip of protruding bone at inner ankle, on posterior edge of tibia.	Branch of saphenous nerve, great saphenous vein.
LV-7	Xi Guan - Knee Joint	Seul Gwan Shitsu Kan	Inner knee, below protruding tibia bone, in head of gastrocnemius m., 1 unit posterior to SP-9.	Branch of medial sural cutaneous nerve, tibial nerve (deeper), posterior tibial artery (deeper).
• LV-8	Qu Quan - Spring at the Bend	Gog Cheon Kyoku Sen	Inner knee joint. When bent, point is at medial end of crease, above tendons attaching at joint.	Saphenous nerve; great saphenous vein, on the path of genu suprema artery (anterior).
LV-9	Yin Bao - Yin Bladder	Eum Po Im Po	4 units above protruding femur bone at inner knee, between vastus medialis m. + sartorius m.	Anterior femoral cutaneous nerve, on pathway of anterior branch of obturator nerve. Deeper+lateral: femoral a. and v., superficial branch of medial circumflex femoral a.
LV-10	(Zu) Wu Li - (Foot) Five Li	(Jog) Gag Ri (Ashi) Go Ri	Upper thigh, 3 units below ST-30, on front edge of adductor longus muscle, where pulse is felt.	Genitofemoral nerve, anterior femoral cutaneous nerve, anterior branch of obturator nerve (deeper), superficial branches of medial circumflex femoral artery and vein.
LV-11	Yin Lian - Yin Corner	Eum Ryeom In Ren	Upper thigh, 2 units below ST-30, on front edge of adductor longus muscle, where pulse is felt.	Genitofemoral nerve, branch of medial femoral cutaneous nerve, anterior branch of obturator nerve (deeper), branches of medial circumflex femoral artery and vein.
• LV-12	Ji Mai - Urgent Pulse	Geub Maeg Kyu Myaku	Inguinal groove, 2.5 units lateral to midline, lateral to pubic symphysis, lateral + below ST-30.	Ilioinguinal n., anterior branch of obturator n. (deeper+inferior), branches of external pudendal a. and v., pubic branches of inferior epigastric a. and v., femoral v. (lateral).
• LV-13	Zhang Men - Camphorwood Gate	Jang Mun Sho Mon	Trunk, below free end of 11th floating rib, 2 units above level of navel, 6 units lateral to midline.*	10th intercostal nerve, 10th intercostal artery and vein. *Note: LV-13 is approximately located where tip of bent elbow touches the trunk.
• LV-14	Qi Men - Cycle Gate	Gi Mun Ki Mon	Chest, near medial end of 6th intercostal space (between ribs), 2 ribs below nipple.*	6th intercostal nerve, 6th intercostal artery and vein. *Note: LV-14 is approximately 3.5 units lateral to CO-14, and 6 units above navel.

Conception (CO)

Primary Paths

The Conception meridian has two primary paths. The first begins in the pelvic cavity, connects to the internal urogenital organs and surfaces in the perineum at CO-1 (between the anus and genitals). It ascends externally up the front midline of the trunk to the chin (CO-24). Here it splits into two internal branches that encircle the mouth and ascend to the area below the eye (ST-1). The second path originates in the pelvic cavity, enters the spine and ascends internally up the back. The Conception meridian intersects the Governing meridian at GV-28.

Function

This meridian regulates the six Regular yin meridians, and is associated with the Liver, Kidneys and uterus.

Key Data

Type:	Yin
Acupoints:	24
Qi-Flow:	Anytime
Related meridian:	Governing

Special Points

Connecting-Luo:	CO-15
Meeting-Hui (Qi):	CO-17
(Yang Organs):	CO-12

Intersection-Jiaohui Points

Stomach —	CO-12, 13, 24
Spleen ---	CO-3, 4, 10, 17
Small Intestine —	CO-12, 13, 17
Kidney ---	CO-3, 4, 17
Pericardium ---	CO-3, 4
Triple Warmer —	CO-12, 17
Liver ---	CO-2, 3, 4
Governing —	CO-1
Penetrating ---	CO-1, 7
Yin Linking ---	CO-22, 23

Points intersecting Conception:
ST-1, GV-28

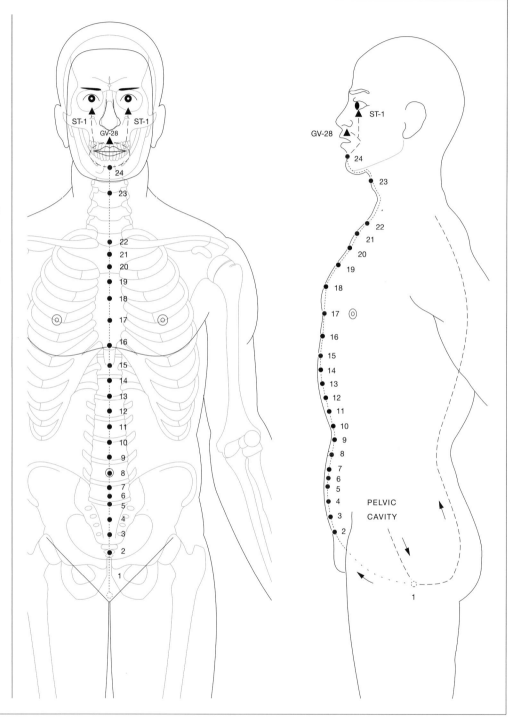

Symbol	Chinese Name	Korean Japanese	Location	Local Anatomy (Nerves and Blood Vessels)
• CO-1	Hui Yin - Meeting of Yin	Hoe Eum E In	In center of perineum, between anus and genitals.	Branch of perineal nerve, branches of perineal artery and vein.

Symbol	Chinese Name	Korean Japanese	Location	Local Anatomy (Nerves and Blood Vessels)
• CO-2	Qu Gu - Curved Bone	Gog Gol Kyoku Kotsu	Front midline, directly above pubic bone (pubic symphysis), 5 units below navel, (pulse is felt).	Branch of iliohypogastric nerve, branches of inferior epigastric artery and obturator artery.
• CO-3	Zhong Ji - Central Pole	Jung Geug Chu Kyoku	Front midline, 1 units above upper edge of pubic bone (pubic symphysis), 4 units below navel.	Branch of iliohypogastric nerve, branches of superficial epigastric and inferior epigastric arteries and veins.
• CO-4	Guan Yuan - Origin Pass	Gwan Weon Kan Gen	Front midline of abdomen, 3 units below navel.	Anterior cutaneous nerve of subcostal nerve, branches of superficial epigastric and inferior epigastric arteries and veins.
• CO-5	Shi Men - Stone Gate	Seog Mun Seki Mon	Front midline of abdomen, 2 units below navel.	Anterior cutaneous branch of 11th intercostal nerve, branches of superficial epigastric and inferior epigastric arteries and veins.
• CO-6	Qi Hai - Sea of Qi	Gi Hae Ki Kai	Front midline of abdomen, 1.5 units below navel.	See CO-5.
CO-7	Yin Jiao - Yin Intersection	Eum Gyo In Ko	Front midline of abdomen, 1 unit below navel.	Anterior cutaneous branch of 10th intercostal nerve, branches of superficial epigastric and inferior epigastric arteries and veins.
• CO-8	Shen Que - Spirit Tower Gate	Sin Gweol Shin Ketsu	Front midline of abdomen, in center of navel.	Anterior cutaneous branch of 10th intercostal nerve, inferior epigastric artery and vein.
CO-9	Shui Fen - Water Divide	Su Bun Sui Bun	Front midline of abdomen, 1 unit above navel.	See CO-8.
CO-10	Xia Wan - Lower Venter	Ha Wan Ge Kan	Front midline of abdomen, 2 units above navel.	See CO-8.
CO-11	Jian Li - Interior Strengthening	Geon Ri Ken Ri	Front midline of abdomen, 3 units above navel.	Anterior cutaneous branch of 8th intercostal nerve, branches of superior epigastric and inferior epigastric arteries and veins.
CO-12	Zhong Wan - Central Venter	Jung Wan Chu Kan	Front midline of abdomen, 4 units above navel.	Anterior cutaneous branch of 7th intercostal nerve, superior epigastric artery and vein.
CO-13	Shang Wan - Upper Venter	Sang Wan Jo Kan	Front midline of abdomen, 5 units above navel.	See CO-12.
CO-14	Ju Que - Great Tower Gate	Geo Gweol Ko Ketsu	Front midline of abdomen, 6 units above navel.	See CO-12.
• CO-15	Jiu Wei - Turtledove Tail	Gu Mi Kyu Bi	Front midline, 7 units above navel, usually below xiphoid process (depends on length of cartilage).	See CO-12.
CO-16	Zhong Ting - Central Palace	Jung Jeong Chu Tei	Front midline, level with 5th intercostal space, in recess where xiphoid process joins sternum.	Anterior cutaneous branch of 6th intercostal nerve, perforating branches of internal mammary artery and vein.
• CO-17	Shan Zhong - Chest Center	Jeon Jung Dan Chu	Front midline of chest, level with 4th intercostal space, level and between nipples, on sternum.	Anterior cutaneous branch of 4th intercostal nerve, perforating branches of internal mammary artery and vein.
CO-18	Yu Tang - Jade Hall	Og Dang Gyoku Do	Front midline of chest, level with 3rd intercostal space, in recess on sternum.	Anterior cutaneous branch of 3rd intercostal nerve, perforating branches of internal mammary artery and vein.
CO-19	Zi Gong - Purple Palace	Ja Gung Shi Kyu	Front midline of chest, level with 2nd intercostal space, in recess on sternum.	Anterior cutaneous branch of 2nd intercostal nerve, perforating branches of internal mammary artery and vein.
CO-20	Hua Gai - Florid Canopy	Wha Gae Ka Gai	Front midline of chest, level with 1st intercostal space, in recess on upper sternum (manubrium).	Anterior cutaneous branch of 1st intercostal nerve, perforating branches of internal mammary artery and vein.
CO-21	Xuan Ji - Jade Pivot	Seon Gi Sen Ki	Front midline, halfway between CO-20 and 22, in recess at center of upper sternum (manubrium).	Medial supraclavicular nerve, anterior cutaneous branch of 1st intercostal nerve, perforating branches of internal mammary artery and vein.
• CO-22	Tian Tu - Celestial Chimney	Cheon Dol Ten Totsu	Front midline, at center of sternal notch (top edge of sternum, at base of throat).	Jugular arch and branch of inferior thyroid artery (near surface), trachea (deeper), inominate vein and aortic arch (inferior and behind sternum).
• CO-23	Lian Quan - Ridge Spring	Yeom Cheon Ren Sen	Front midline of throat, above Adam's apple, in recess at upper edge of hyoid bone.	Branch of cutaneous cervical nerve, hypoglossal nerve, branch of glossopharyngeal nerve, anterior jugular vein.
• CO-24	Cheng Jiang - Sauce Receptacle	Seung Jang Sho Sho	Front midline of jaw, in center of groove between chin and lower lip (mentolabial groove).	Branch of facial nerve, branches of inferior labial artery and vein.

Governing (GV)

Primary Paths

The Governing meridian has four paths. The first begins in the pelvic cavity, surfaces in the perineum at CO-1, and ascends externally up the midline of the spine to GV-16 at the back of the neck. It then enters the brain, surfaces at the vertex (GV-20), and descends the forehead to end at the upper gum. The second path begins in the pelvic area and ascends the spine to the Kidneys. The third path (bilateral) begins at the inner corner of both eyes (BL-1), converges at the vertex, descends through the brain to emerge at the back-lower neck. Here it redivides into two paths that descend opposite sides of the spine to join the Kidneys. The fourth path begins in the lower abdomen, ascends through the Heart and trachea, and divides into two branches that encircle the mouth and end below the eyes.

Function

The Governing meridian regulates the six Regular yang meridians, which meet at GV-14. This meridian is associated with the physiology of the brain, spine and reproductive organs.

Key Data

Type: Yang
Acupoints: 28
Qi-Flow: Anytime
Related meridian: Conception

Special Points

Connecting-Luo: GV-1

Intersection-Jiaohui Points

Large Intestine — GV-14, 26
Stomach —   GV-14, 24, 26
Small Intestine — GV-14
Bladder —   GV-13, 14, 17, 20, 24
Kidney ---   GV-1
Triple Warmer —   GV-14
Gallbladder —   GV-1, GV-14
Conception —   GV-28
Yang Linking —   GV-15, 16
Yang Heel —   GV-16

Points intersecting Governing:
BL-12, CO-1

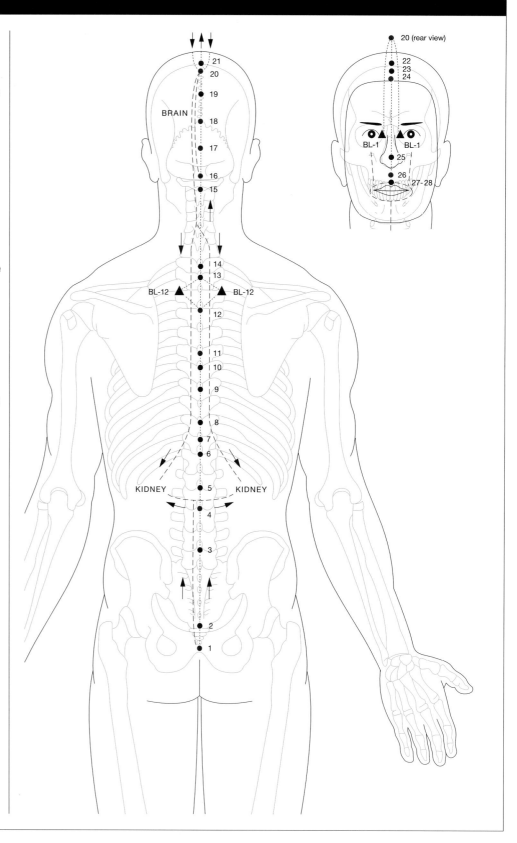

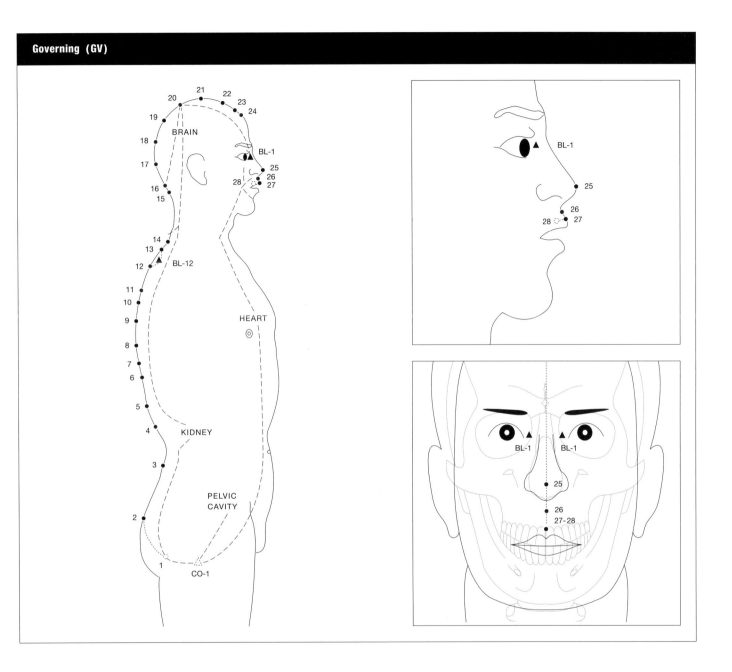

Symbol	Chinese Name	Korean Japanese	Location	Local Anatomy (Nerves and Blood Vessels)
• GV-1	Chang Qiang - Long Strong	Jang Gang Cho Kyo	Halfway between tip of tailbone (coccyx) and anus.	Posterior ramus of coccygeal nerve, hemorrhoid nerve, branches of inferior hemorrhoid artery and vein.
GV-2	Yao Shu - Lumbar Shu	Yo Yu Yo Yu	Rear midline, at sacral hiatus.	Branch of coccygeal nerve, branches of median sacral artery and vein.
GV-3	(Yao) Yang Guan - (Lumbar) Yang Pass	Yang Gwan Yo Kan	Midline of back, below spinous process of 4th lumbar vertebra.	Medial branch of posterior ramus of lumbar nerve, posterior branch of lumbar artery.
• GV-4	Ming Men - Life Gate	Myeong Mun Mei Mon	Midline of back, below spinous process of 2nd lumbar vertebra.	See GV-3.
GV-5	Xuan Shu - Suspended Pivot	Hyeon Chu Ken Su	Midline of back, below spinous process of 1st lumbar vertebra.	See GV-3.

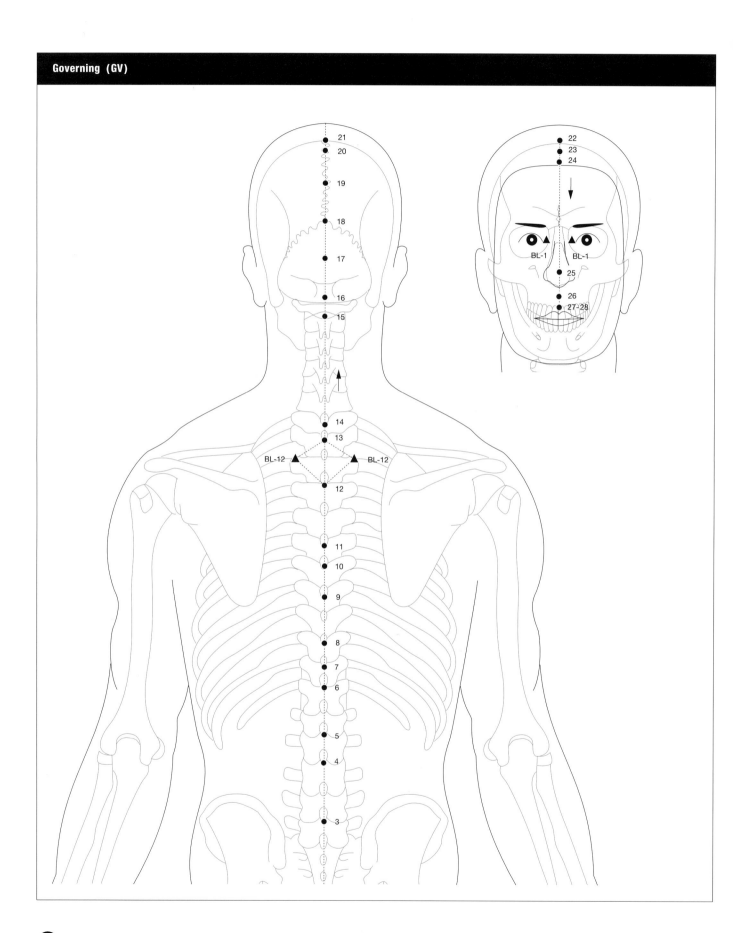

Symbol	Chinese Name	Korean Japanese	Location	Local Anatomy (Nerves and Blood Vessels)
GV-6	Ji Zhong - Spinal Center	Cheog Jung Seki Chu	Midline of back, below spinous process of 11th thoracic vertebra.	Medial branch of posterior ramus of 11th thoracic nerve, posterior branch of 11th intercostal artery.
GV-7	Zhong Shu - Central Pivot	Jung Chu Chu Su	Midline of back, below spinous process of 10th thoracic vertebra.	Medial branch of posterior ramus of 10th thoracic nerve, posterior branch of 10th intercostal artery.
GV-8	Jin Suo - Sinew Contraction	Geun Chug Kin Shuku	Midline of back, below spinous process of 9th thoracic vertebra.	Medial branch of posterior ramus of 9th thoracic nerve, posterior branch of 9th intercostal artery.
GV-9	Zhi Yang - Extremity of Yang	Ji Yang Shi Yo	Midline of back, below spinous process of 7th thoracic vertebra, about level to base of scapula.	Medial branch of posterior ramus of 7th thoracic nerve, posterior branch of 7th intercostal artery.
GV-10	Ling Tai - Spirit Tower	Yeong Dae Rei Dai	Midline of back, below spinous process of 6th thoracic vertebra.	Medial branch of posterior ramus of 6th thoracic nerve, posterior branch of 6th intercostal artery.
• GV-11	Shen Dao - Spirit Path	Sin Do Shin Do	Midline of back, below spinous process of 5th thoracic vertebra.	Medial branch of posterior ramus of 5th thoracic nerve, posterior branch of 5th intercostal artery.
• GV-12	Shen Zhu - Body Pillar	Sin Ju Shin Chu	Midline of back, below spinous process of 3rd thoracic vertebra.	Medial branch of posterior ramus of 3rd thoracic nerve, posterior branch of 3rd intercostal artery.
GV-13	Tao Dao - Kiln Path	Do Do To Do	Midline of back, below spinous process of 1st thoracic vertebra.	Medial branch of posterior ramus of 1st thoracic nerve, posterior branch of 1st intercostal artery.
GV-14	Da Zhui - Great Hammer	Dae Toe Dai Tsui	Midline at level of shoulder, between spinous processes of 7th cervical+1st thoracic vertebras.	Posterior ramus of 8th cervical nerve, medial branch of posterior ramus of 1st thoracic nerve, branch of transverse cervical artery.
• GV-15	Ya Men - Mute's Gate	A Mun A Mon	Back midline of neck, in recess 0.5 unit below GV-16, 0.5 unit within hairline.	3rd occipital nerve, branches of occipital artery and vein.
• GV-16	Feng Fu - Wind Mansion	Pung Bu Fu Fu	Midline of neck, in recess below ext. occipital protuberance, at trapezius muscle attachments.	Branches of 3rd occipital nerve and great occipital nerve, branch of occipital artery.
• GV-17	Nao Hu - Brain's Door	Noe Ho No Ko	Back midline of head, 1.5 units above GV-16, above external occipital protuberance (bone).	Branch of great occipital nerve, branches of occipital arteries and veins of both sides.
• GV-18	Qiang Jian - Unyielding Space	Gang Gan Kyo Kan	Back midline of head, 1.5 units above GV-17, halfway between GV-16 and GV-20.	See GV-17.
GV-19	Hou Ding - Behind the Vertex	Hu Jeong Go Cho	Back midline of head, 1.5 units above (anterior) GV-18, or 1.5 units posterior to GV-20.	See GV-17.
• GV-20	Bai Hui - Hundred Convergences	Baeg Hae Hyaku E	Midline of head, 7 units above rear hairline, on midpoint of line joining earlobes and ear apexes.	Branch of great occipital nerve, anastomotic network formed by superficial temporal arteries and veins and occipital arteries and veins of both sides.
GV-21	Qian Ding - Before the Vertex	Jeon Jeong Zen Cho	Midline, on top of head, 1.5 units in front of (anterior) GV-20.	On communicating site of branch of frontal nerve with branch of great occipital nerve, anastomotic network formed by left and right superficial temporal arteries and veins.
GV-22	Xin Hui - Fontanel Meeting	Sin Hoe Shin E	Midline, on top of head, 3 units in front of (anterior) GV-20, 2 units within front hairline.	Branch of frontal nerve, anastomotic network formed by superficial temporal artery and vein and frontal artery and vein.
GV-23	Shang Xing - Upper Star	Sang Seong Jo Sei	Midline, on top of head, 4 units in front of (anterior) GV-20, 1 unit within front hairline.	Branch of frontal nerve, branches of superficial temporal artery and vein, branches of frontal artery and vein.
• GV-24	Shen Ting - Spirit Court	Sin Jeong Shin Tei	Midline, on top of head, 0.5 unit within front hairline.	Branch of frontal nerve, branches of frontal artery and vein.
GV-25	Su Liao - White Bone-Hole	So Ryo So Ryo	Front midline, at very tip of nose.	External nasal branch of anterior ethmoid nerve, nasal branch of facial artery and vein.
• GV-26	Shui Gou - Water Trough Ren Zhong - Human Ctr.	Su Gu Sui Ko	Front midline, in center of groove below nose (philtrum), slightly above midpoint.	Buccal branch of facial nerve, branch of infraorbital nerve, superior labial artery and vein.
GV-27	Dui Duan - Extremity of Mouth	Tae Dan Da Tan	Front midline, at peak of upper lip, where upper lip meets philtrum.	See GV-26.
GV-28	Yin Jiao - Gum Intersection	Eun Gyo Gin Ko	Front midline, in cleft above teeth on gum (frenulum of upper lip).	Branch of superior alveolar nerve, superior labial artery and vein.

Penetrating

Primary Paths

The Penetrating meridian has five paths. The first begins in the lower abdomen, surfaces in the perineum at CO-1, intersects ST-30, ascends externally up the abdomen along the Kidney meridian (also intersecting CO-7), and ends in the chest region, where it disperses Qi. The second path begins in the chest, where the first path disperses: it ascends the throat and face, encircles the mouth, and ends in the nasal cavity. The third path begins in the lower abdomen, descends the inner leg, and passes behind the protruding bone at ankle, ending in the sole of the foot. The fourth path separates from the third path along the tibia (lower leg), enters the heel and crosses the foot, ending at the big toe. The fifth path separates from the main path in the pelvic cavity and ascends the spine.

Function

The Penetrating meridian has a regulating effect on all 12 Regular meridians, and is associated with menstruation and the physiology of the reproductive organs. The Penetrating meridian is also considered an important link between the Kidney and Stomach meridians, and between the Conception and Governing meridians.

Key Data

Type:	Yin
Bilateral Acupoints:	12 (x2)
Midline Acupoints:	2
Qi-Flow:	Anytime
Related meridian:	Girdling

Special Acupoints

Confluence-Jiaohui: SP-4

Intersection Points with other Extraordinary meridians
Conception —   CO-1, 7

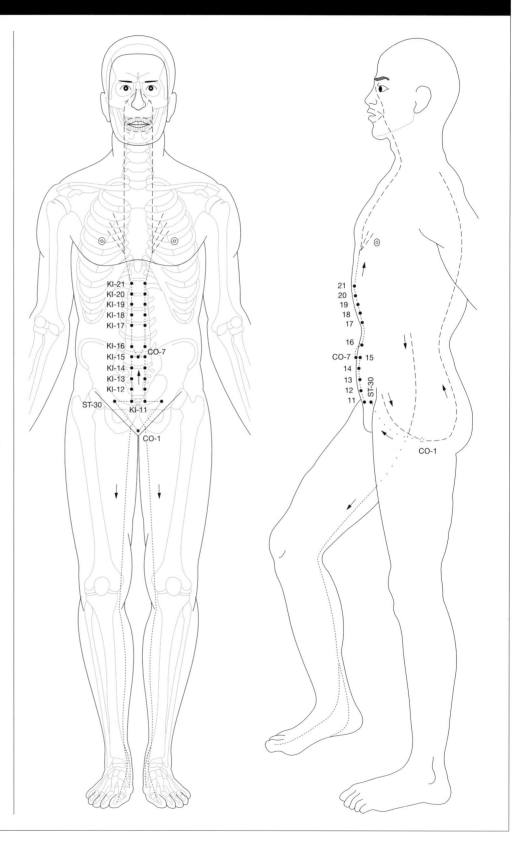

Penetrating

Symbol	Chinese Name	Korean Japanese	Location	Local Anatomy (Nerves and Blood Vessels)
• CO-1	Hui Yin - Meeting of Yin	Hoe Eum E In	In center of perineum, between anus and genitals.	Branch of perineal nerve, branches of perineal artery and vein.
CO-7	Yin Jiao - Yin Intersection	Eum Gyo In Ko	Front midline of abdomen, 1 unit below navel.	Anterior cutaneous branch of 10th intercostal nerve, branches of superficial epigastric and inferior epigastric arteries and veins.
KI-11	Heng Gu - Pubic Bone	Hoeng Gol O Kotsu	In moon-shaped recess 5 units below navel, at upper edge of pubic bone, 0.5 unit lateral CO-2.	Branch of iliohypogastric nerve, inferior epigastric artery and external pudendal artery.
KI-12	Da He - Great Manifestation	Dae Hyeog Tai Kaku	Abdomen, 4 units below navel, 0.5 unit lateral CO-3.	Branches of subcostal nerve and iliohypogastric nerve, muscular branches of inferior epigastric artery and vein.
KI-13	Qi Xue - Qi Hole	Gi Hyeol Ki Ketsu	Abdomen, 3 units below navel, 0.5 unit lateral CO-4.	See KI-12.
KI-14	Si Man - Fourfold Fullness	Sa Man Shi Man	Abdomen, 2 units below navel, 0.5 unit lateral CO-5.	See KI-12.
KI-15	Zhong Zhu - Central Flow	Jung Ju Chu Chu	Abdomen, 1 unit below navel, 0.5 unit lateral CO-7.	10th intercostal nerve, muscular branches of inferior epigastric artery and vein.
KI-16	Huang Shu - Vital Shu	Hwang Yu Ko Yu	Abdomen, 0.5 unit lateral to center of navel (CO-8).	10th intercostal nerve, muscular branches of inferior epigastric artery and vein.
KI-17	Shang Qu - Shang Bend	Seog Gwan Sho Kyoku	Abdomen, 2 units above navel, 0.5 unit lateral CO-10.	9th intercostal nerve, branches of superior and inferior epigastric artery and vein.
KI-18	Shi Guan - Stone Pass	Sang Gog Seki Kan	Abdomen, 3 units above navel, 0.5 unit lateral CO-11.	8th intercostal nerve, branches of superior epigastric artery and vein.
KI-19	Yin Du - Yin Metropolis	Eum Do In To	Abdomen, 4 units above navel, 0.5 unit lateral CO-12.	See KI-18.
KI-20	Tong Gu - Open Valley	Tong Gog (Bok) Tsu Koku	Abdomen, 5 units above navel, 0.5 unit lateral CO-13.	See KI-18.
KI-21	You Men - Dark Gate	Yu Mun Yu Mon	Abdomen, 6 units above navel, 0.5 unit lateral CO-14.	7th intercostal nerve, branches of superior epigastric artery and vein.
ST-30	Qi Chong - Surging Qi	Gi Chung Ki Sho	5 units below navel, 2 units lateral to CO-2, above inguinal groove, medial side of femoral a.	Path of Ilioinguinal nerve, branches of superficial epigastric artery and vein, inferior epigastric artery and vein (slightly lateral), femoral artery (pulse is felt).

Girdling

Primary Paths

The Girdling meridian begins below the hypochondrium (upper-outer part of the abdomen) at the level of the second lumbar vertebra, and below the lateral tip of the tenth rib. This meridian circles the waist like a "belt" or "girdle," intersecting the Gallbladder meridian at GB-26, GB-27 and GB-28. Most healing arts define the Girdling meridian as composed of these three bilateral acupoints. Some healing arts also include LV-13, which is sometimes defined as the origin of the meridian. If LV-13 is included, the Girdling meridian consists of four bilateral acupoints.

Function

The Girdling meridian has a regulating effect on the flow of Qi, in all the meridians that run up and down the trunk. It is associated with the physiology of the lumbar region, abdomen, lower limbs, and female reproductive system.

Key Data

Type: Yang
Acupoints: 3 (x2)
Qi-Flow: Anytime
Related meridian: Penetrating

Special Points

Confluence-Jiaohui: GB-41

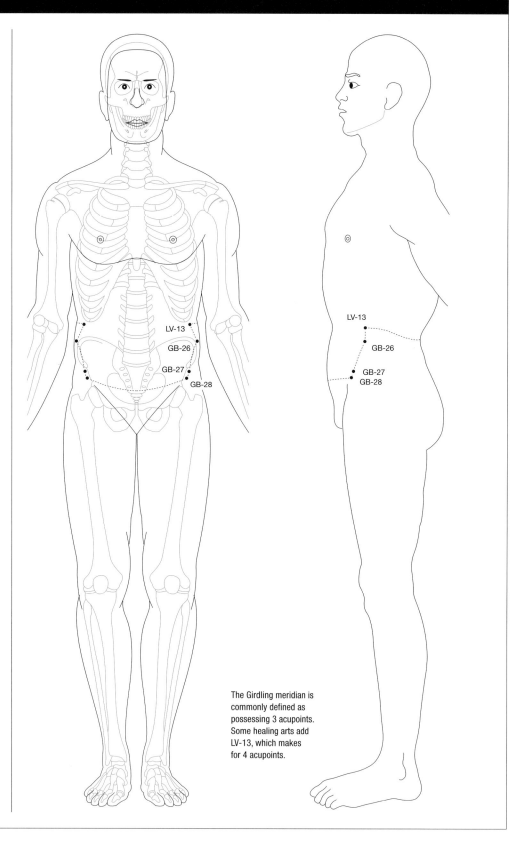

LV-13
GB-26
GB-27
GB-28

LV-13
GB-26
GB-27
GB-28

The Girdling meridian is commonly defined as possessing 3 acupoints. Some healing arts add LV-13, which makes for 4 acupoints.

Girdling

Symbol	Chinese Name	Korean Japanese	Location	Local Anatomy (Nerves and Blood Vessels)
GB-26	Dai Mai - Girdling Vessel	Dae Maeg Tai Myaku	Side of trunk, level with navel, vertically aligned with free end of 11th floating rib (LV-13).	Subcostal nerve, subcostal artery and vein.
GB-27	Wu Shu - Fifth Pivot	O Chu Go Su	Abdomen, on anterior side of front-upper iliac spine of hipbone, 3 units below level of navel.	Iliohypogastric nerve, superficial and deep circumflex iliac arteries and veins.
GB-28	Wei Dao - Linking Path	Yu Do Yui Do	0.5 unit below and slightly medial to GB-27, slightly below front-upper iliac spine of hipbone.	Ilioinguinal nerve, superficial and deep circumflex iliac arteries and veins.
• LV-13	Zhang Men - Camphorwood Gate	Jang Mun Sho Mon	Trunk, below free end of 11th floating rib, 2 units above level of navel, 6 units lateral to midline.*	10th intercostal nerve, 10th intercostal artery and vein. *Note: LV-13 is approximately located where tip of bent elbow touches the trunk.

Yin Linking

Primary Paths

The Yin Linking meridian begins on the inner surface of the lower leg at KI-9. This area is also common to all three of the Leg-Yin Meridians: the Spleen, Liver and Kidney. From KI-9, the Yin Linking meridian ascends along the inner leg and abdomen, intersecting acupoints on the Spleen and Liver meridians. It continues up the chest to the throat, where it intersects the Conception meridian at CO-22 and CO-23.

Function

The Yin Linking meridian has a regulating effect on the Qi-flows in the six Regular yin meridians: the Lung, Spleen, Heart, Kidney, Pericardium and Liver. The Yin Linking meridian is said to control the "nourishing" energy of the body, and regulates the Blood and interior regions. Whereas, the Yang Linking meridian is associated with exterior regions.

Key Data

Type: Yin
Bilateral Acupoints: 6 (x2)
Midline Acupoints: 2
Qi-Flow: Anytime
Related meridian: Yang Linking

Special Points

Confluence-Jiaohui: PC-6

Intersection Points with other
Extraordinary meridians
Conception —   CO-22, 23

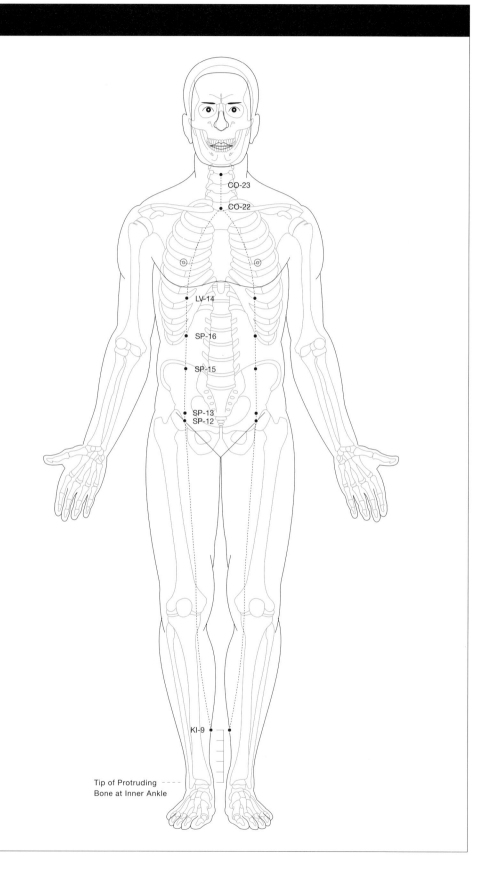

Symbol	Chinese Name	Korean Japanese	Location	Local Anatomy (Nerves and Blood Vessels)
• CO-22	Tian Tu - Celestial Chimney	Cheon Dol Ten Totsu	Front midline, at center of sternal notch (top edge of sternum, at base of throat).	Jugular arch and branch of inferior thyroid artery (near surface), trachea (deeper), inominate vein and aortic arch (inferior and behind sternum).
• CO-23	Lian Quan - Ridge Spring	Yeom Cheon Ren Sen	Front midline of throat, above Adam's apple, in recess at upper edge of hyoid bone.	Branch of cutaneous cervical nerve, hypoglossal nerve, branch of glossopharyngeal nerve, anterior jugular vein.
KI-9	Zhu Bin - Guest House	Chug Bin Chiku Hin	Inner lower leg, at lower inner edge of body of gastrocnemius m. (calf), 5 units above KI-3.	Medial sural cutaneous nerve, and medial crural cutaneous nerve, tibial nerve (deeper), posterior tibial artery and vein (deeper).
• LV-14	Qi Men - Cycle Gate	Gi Mun Ki Mon	Chest, near medial end of 6th intercostal space (between ribs), 2 ribs below nipple.*	6th intercostal nerve, 6th intercostal artery and vein. *Note: LV-14 is approximately 3.5 units lateral to CO-14, and 6 units above navel.
• SP-12	Chong Men - Surging Gate	Chung Mun Sho Mon	In inguinal crease, lateral side of femoral artery, 3.5 units lateral to CO-2, where pulse is felt.	Point where femoral nerve traverses, femoral artery (on medial side).
SP-13	Fu She - Bowel Abode	Bu Sa Fu Sha	Abdomen, 0.7 unit above SP-12, 3.5 units lateral to body midline.	Ilioinguinal nerve.
SP-15	Da Heng - Great Horizontal	Dae Hoeng Dai O	Abdomen, 3.5 units lateral to center of navel, at lateral edge of rectus abdominus muscle.	10th intercostal nerve, 10th intercostal artery and vein.
SP-16	Fu Ai - Abdominal Lament	Bog Ae Fuku Ai	Abdomen, 3 units above SP-15. 3.5 units lateral to body midline.	8th intercostal nerve, 8th intercostal artery and vein.

Yang Linking

Primary Paths

The Yang Linking meridian begins on the outer foot, below the protruding bone of outer ankle, at BL-63. This area is also common to all three of the Leg-Yang Meridians: the Stomach, Gallbladder and Bladder. From BL-63, it ascends the outer leg along the path of the Gallbladder meridian, intersecting GB-35. It continues to climb the outer back, up to the rear of the shoulder, where it intersects SI-10. From here, it ascends the neck, passes behind the ear to the forehead, returns back over the top of the head, and descends to the top of the back of the neck, ending at GV-16. During its route, the Yang Linking meridian intersects acupoints on the Bladder, Gallbladder, Small Intestine, Triple Warmer and Governing meridians.

Function

The Yang Linking meridian has a regulating effect on the Qi-flows in the six Regular yang meridians: the Large Intestine, Stomach, Small Intestine, Bladder, Triple Warmer and Gallbladder. The Yang Linking meridian is said to control the "defensive" energy of the body and resistance to external pathogens (causes of disease), and regulates the exterior regions. Whereas, the Yin Linking meridian is associated with interior regions.

Key Data

Type:	Yang
Bilateral Acupoints:	13 (x2)
Midline Acupoints:	2
Qi-Flow:	Anytime
Related meridian:	Yin Linking

Special Points

Confluence-Jiaohui: TW-5

*Intersection Points with other
Extraordinary meridians*

Governing —	GV-15, 16
Yang Heel —	GB-20

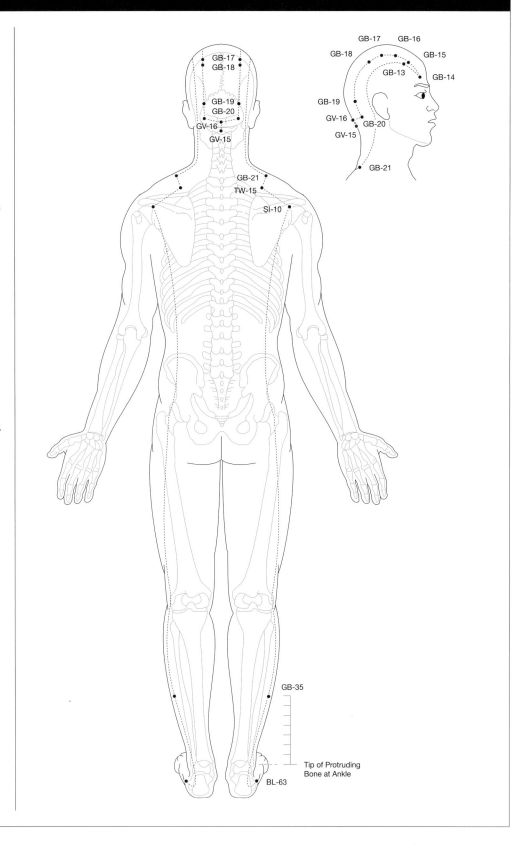

Symbol	Chinese Name	Korean Japanese	Location	Local Anatomy (Nerves and Blood Vessels)
BL-63	Jin Men - Metal Gate	Geum Mun Kim Mon	Outer foot, in recess below cuboid bone, forward and down (anterior and inferior) from BL-62.	Lateral dorsal cutaneous nerve of foot, lateral plantar nerve (deeper), lateral plantar artery and vein.
• GB-13	Ben Shen - Root Spirit	Bon Sin Hon Jin	3 units lateral to GV-24, 0.5 unit within hairline of forehead, 2/3 the distance from GV-24 to ST-8.	Lateral branch of frontal nerve, frontat branches of superficial temporal artery and vein, lateral branches of frontal artery and vein.
• GB-14	Yang Bai - Yang White	Yang Baek Yo Haku	Forehead, 1 unit above midpoint of eyebrow, aligned with eye pupil.	Lateral branch of frontal nerve, lateral branches of frontal artery and vein.
• GB-15	Tou Lin Qi - Head Overlooking Tears	Im Eub Atama Rin Kyu	Forehead, directly above GB-14, 0.5 unit within hairline, halfway between GV-24 and ST-8.	Anastomotic branch of medial and lateral branches of frontal nerve, frontal artery and vein.
• GB-16	Mu Chuang - Eye Window	Mog Chang Moku So	Head, 1.5 units posterior to GB-15, on line joining GB-15 to GB-20.	Anastomotic branch of medial and lateral branches of frontal nerve, frontal branches of superficial temporal artery and vein.
• GB-17	Zheng Ying - Upright Construction	Jeong Yeong Sho Ei	Head, 1.5 units posterior to GB-16, on line joining GB-15 to GB-20.	Anastomotic branch of frontal and great occipital nerves, anastomotic plexus formed by parietal branches of superficial temporal artery and vein and occipital a. and v.
• GB-18	Cheng Ling - Spirit Support	Seung Lyeong Sho Rei	On head, 1.5 units posterior to GB-17, on line joining GB-15 to GB-20.	Branch of great auricular nerve, branches of occipital artery and vein.
GB-19	Nao Kong - Brain Hollow	Noe Gong No Ku	Back of head, directly above GB-20, level with GV-17, lateral side of protruding occipital bone.	See GB-18.
• GB-20	Feng Chi - Wind Pool	Pung Ji Fu Chi	Back of neck, below occipital bone, in recess between sternoceidomastoid m. and trapezius m.	Branch of lesser occipital nerve, branches of occipital artery and vein.
• GB-21	Jian Jing - Shoulder Well	Gyeon Jeong Ken Sei	Shoulder, halfway between C7 vertebra and protruding bone at top of shoulder (acromion).	Lateral branch of supraclavicular nerve, accessory nerve, transverse cervical artery and vein.
GB-35	Yang Jiao - Yang Intersection	Yang Gyo Yo Ko	7 units above protruding bone tip at outer ankle, on rear edge of fibula, level with GB-36 + BL-58.	Lateral sural cutaneous nerve, branches of peroneal artery and vein.
• GV-15	Ya Men - Mute's Gate	A Mun A Mon	Back midline of neck, in recess 0.5 unit below GV-16, 0.5 unit within hairline.	3rd occipital nerve, branches of occipital artery and vein.
• GV-16	Feng Fu - Wind Mansion	Pung Bu Fu Fu	Midline of neck, in recess below ext. occipital protuberance, at trapezius muscle attachments.	Branches of 3rd occipital nerve and great occipital nerve, branch of occipital artery.
SI-10	Nao Shu - Upper Arm Shu	No Yu Ju Yu	Directly above SI-9 when arm is lowered, in recess below scapular spine (ridge).	Posterior cutaneous nerve of arm, axillary nerve, suprascapular nerve (deeper), posterior circumflex humeral artery and vein, subscapular artery and vein (deeper).
• TW-15	Tian Liao - Celestial Bone-Hole	Cheon Ryo Ten Ryo	Above shoulder blade (scapula), halfway between GB-21 and SI-13.	Accessory nerve, branch of suprascapular nerve, descending branch of transverse cervical artery, muscular branch of suprascapular artery (deeper).

Yin Heel

Primary Paths

The Yin Heel meridian (also called the Yin Heel Vessel) begins on the inner foot, just below the protruding bone of inner ankle, at KI-6. It ascends the inner leg, intersects KI-8, crosses the genital region, rises up the chest, and enters the body at the supraclavicular fossa. From here, it ascends internally through the throat, surfaces in front of ST-9, and continues up the cheek, ending at the inner corner of the eye (BL-1). Here it joins the Yang Heel meridian and the Bladder meridian, which ascend over the head and enter the brain.

Function

The Yin Heel and Yang Heel meridians act as a bridge linking yin and yang energies. They primarily control physiologic functions involving the ascent of Fluids and the descent of Qi, the opening and closing of the eyes, and general muscular activity. The Yin Heel meridian is also associated with the physiology of the eye, lower leg muscles, lower abdomen, and genitals.

Key Data

Type:	Yin
Acupoints:	3 (x2)
Qi-Flow:	Anytime
Related meridian:	Yang Heel

Special Points

Confluence-Jiaohui: KI-6

Intersection Points with other Extraordinary meridians
Yang Heel —   BL-1

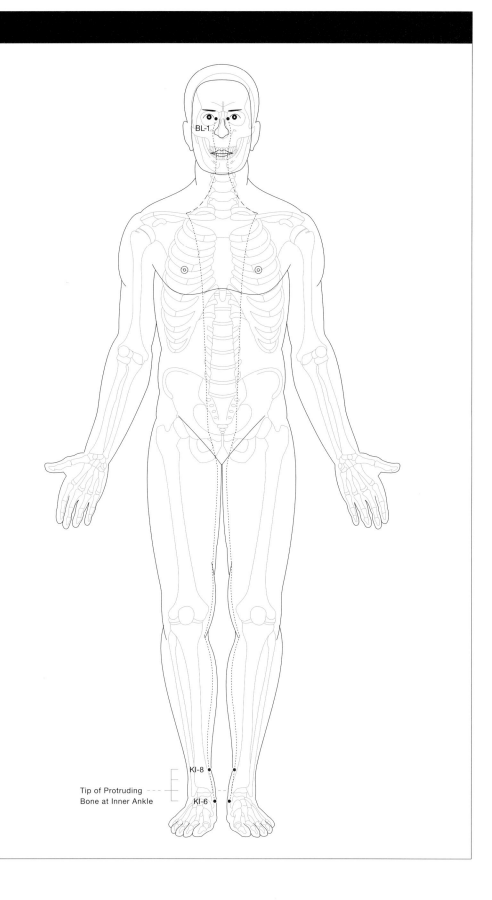

Symbol	Chinese Name	Korean Japanese	Location	Local Anatomy (Nerves and Blood Vessels)
BL-1	Jing Ming - Bright Eyes	Jeong Myeong Sei Mei	0.1 unit above inner corner of eye (inner canthus), located with eyes closed.	Supratrochlear and infratrochlear nerves (near surface), branches of oculomotor nerve (deeper), opthalmic n. (deeper), angular a. and v., opthalmic a. and v. (above, deeper)
KI-6	Zhao Hai - Shining Sea	Jo Hae Sho Kai	Inner side of foot, in recess 1 unit below tip of protruding bone at ankle (medial malleolus).	Medial crural cutaneous nerve, tibial nerve (deeper), posterior tibial artery and vein (slightly posterior and inferior).
KI-8	Jiao Xin - Intersection Reach	Gyo Sin Ko Shin	Inner lower leg, 2 units above KI-3, 0.5 unit anterior to KI-7, behind medial edge of tibia.	Medial crural cutaneous nerves, tibial nerve (deeper), posterior tibial artery and vein (deeper).
			Note: KI-3 is in recess between protruding bone at inner ankle and Achilles tendon, level with tip.	
			Note: KI-7 is in recess on front (anterior) edge of Achilles tendon, 2 units above KI-3.	

Yang Heel

Primary Paths

The Yang Heel meridian (also called the Yang Heel Vessel) begins on the outer foot, below the protruding bone of outer ankle, at BL-62. It ascends the outer leg and side of the torso, passing up to the back of the shoulder. It then crosses the shoulder to the front side of the body, and ascends the neck and cheek to the inner corner of the eye, where it joins the Yin Heel meridian and the Bladder meridian at BL-1. From this point, it continues over the head and descends behind the ear to intersect GB-20, before traversing to the base of the skull, where it enters the brain at GV-16. During its route, the Yang Heel meridian intersects acupoints on the Bladder, Gallbladder, Small Intestine, Large Intestine, Stomach and Governing meridians.

Function

The Yin Heel and Yang Heel meridians act as a bridge linking yin and yang energies. They primarily control physiologic functions involving the ascent of Fluids and the descent of Qi, the opening and closing of the eyes, and general muscular activity. The Yang Heel meridian is also associated with the physiology of the eye, lower leg muscles and lumbar region.

Key Data

Type:	Yang
Bilateral Acupoints:	12 (x2)
Midline Acupoints:	1
Qi-Flow:	Anytime
Related meridian:	Yin Heel

Special Points

Confluence-Jiaohui: BL-62

Intersection Points with other Extraordinary meridians

Yin Heel ---	BL-1
Governing —	GV-16
Yang Linking —	GV-16, GB-20, SI-10

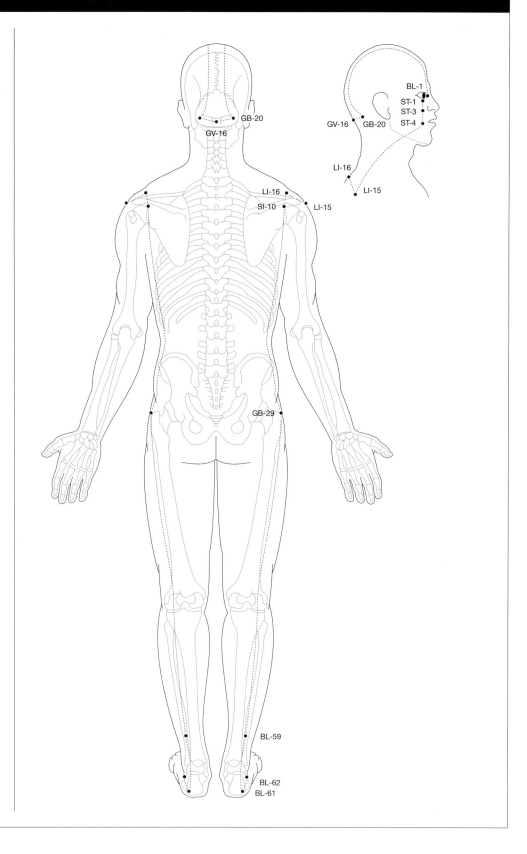

Symbol	Chinese Name	Korean Japanese	Location	Local Anatomy (Nerves and Blood Vessels)
BL-1	Jing Ming - Bright Eyes	Jeong Myeong Sei Mei	0.1 unit above inner corner of eye (inner canthus), located with eyes closed.	Supratrochlear and infratrochlear nerves (near surface), branches of oculomotor nerve (deeper), opthalmic n. (deeper), angular a. and v., opthalmic a. and v. (above, deeper)
BL-59	Fu Yang - Instep Yang	Bu Yang Fu Yo	Lower leg, 3 units directly above BL-60, at lateral side of gastrocnemius muscle.*	Sural nerve, small saphenous vein, terminal branch of peroneal artery (deeper). *Note: BL-59 is located on line joining BL-58 to BL-60.
BL-61	Pu Can - Subservient Visitor	Bog Sam Boku Shin	Outer heel, below BL-60* in recess at heel bone (calcaneus), at edge of red and white skin.	External calcaneal branch of sural nerve, external calcaneal branch of peroneal artery and vein.
BL-62	Shen Mai - Extending Vessel	Sin Maeg Shim Myaku	Outer foot, in recess directly below protruding bone at ankle (external malleolus).	Sural nerve, external malleolar arterial network.
• GB-20	Feng Chi - Wind Pool	Pung Ji Fu Chi	Back of neck, below occipital bone, in recess between sternoceidomastoid m. and trapezius m.	Branch of lesser occipital nerve, branches of occipital artery and vein.
GB-29	Ju Liao - Squating Bone-Hole	Geo Ryo Kyo Ryo	Halfway between front-upper iliac spine of hip-bone + protruding bone at upper leg (trochanter).	Lateral femoral cutaneous nerve, branches of superficial circumflex iliac artery and vein, ascending branches of lateral circumflex femoral artery and vein.
• GV-16	Feng Fu - Wind Mansion	Pung Bu Fu Fu	Midline of neck, in recess below ext. occipital protuberance, at trapezius muscle attachments.	Branches of 3rd occipital nerve and great occipital nerve, branch of occipital artery.
• LI-15	Jian Yu - Shoulder Bone	Gyeon U Ken Gu	With arm raised, in a recess at edge of shoulder joint, slightly forward to middle of deltoid muscle.	Axillary nerve, lateral supraclavicular nerve, posterior circumflex humeral artery and vein.
LI-16	Ju Gu - Great Bone	Geo Gol Ko Kotsu	Top of shoulder, in recess between end of clavicle and scapular spine (between 2 forking bones).	Lateral supraclavicular nerve and branch of accessory nerve (near surface), suprascapular nerve (deeper), jugular vein, suprascapular artery and vein (deeper).
SI-10	Nao Shu - Upper Arm Shu	No Yu Ju Yu	Directly above SI-9** when arm is lowered, in recess below scapular spine (ridge).	Posterior cutaneous nerve of arm, axillary nerve, suprascapular nerve (deeper), posterior circumflex humeral artery and vein, subscapular artery and vein (deeper).
ST-1	Cheng Qi - Tear Container	Seung Eub Sho Kyu	Directly below eye pupil, in recess above cheekbone at lower eyelid.	Branch of intraorbital nerve, inferior branch of oculomotor nerve, muscular branch of facial nerve, branches of infraorbital and ophthalmic arteries and veins.
ST-3	Ju Liao - Great Bone-Hole	Geo Ryo Ko Ryo	Directly below eye pupil and ST-1 and ST-2, level with lower edge of nostril.	Branches of facial and infraorbital nerves, branches of facial and infraorbital arteries and veins.
• ST-4	Di Cang - Earth Granary	Ji Chang Chi So	Slightly lateral to corner of mouth, directly below ST-3, a faint pulse is felt close below.	Branches of facial and infraorbital nerves, terminal branch of buccal nerve (deeper), facial and artery and vein.
			* BL-60 is in recess halfway between protruding bone at ankle and Achilles tendon, level with tip.	
			** SI-9 is on back, below shoulder joint, 1 unit above end of axillary fold when arm is lowered.	

Extra Acupoints

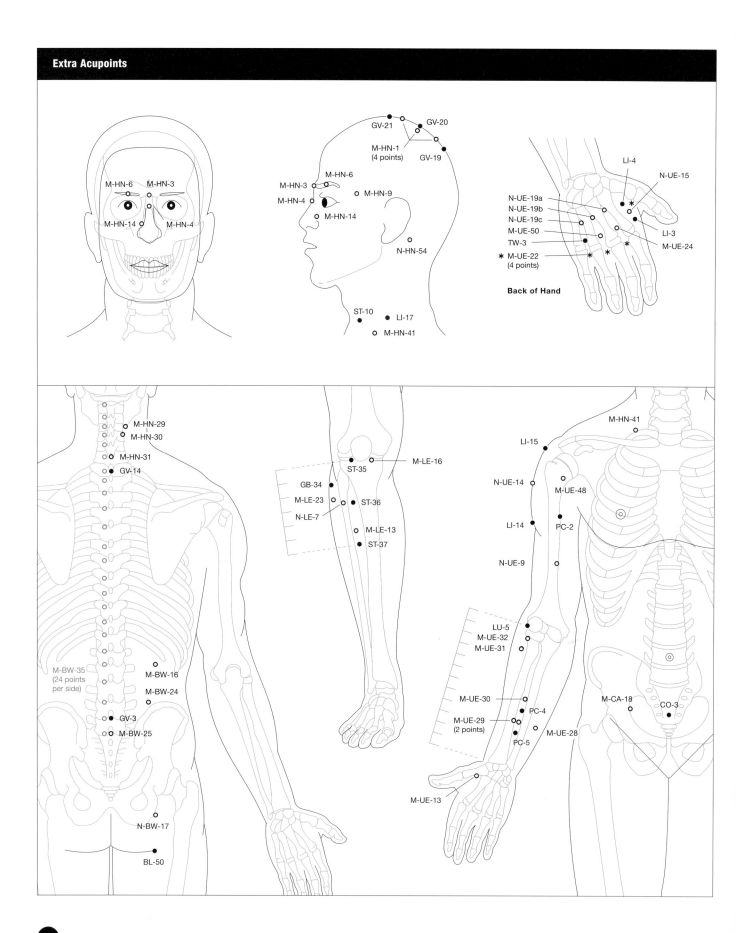

Extra acupoints in this book are identified using the established alphanumeric (letter/number) system employed by O'Connor and Bensky. The first letter refers to the acupoint category: M = Miscellaneous or N = New. Subsequent letters refer to general body location as outlined at right. Of the 394-plus Extra acupoints identified, only those commonly used in martial and healing applications are outlined below and on the next two pages. Comprehensive acupuncture texts will list additional Extra acupoints.

M	Miscellaneous Acupoint	HN	Head and Neck
N	New Acupoint	CA	Chest and Abdomen
		BW	Back and Waist
		UE	Upper Extremity
		LE	Lower Extremity

Symbol	Chinese Name	Location	Local Anatomy (Nerves and Blood Vessels)
M-BW-16	Pi Gen - Lump's Root	Lower back, 3.5 units lateral to lower edge of spinous process of 1st lumbar vertebra.	
M-BW-24	Yao Yan - Lumbar Eye	Lower back, in recess 3–4 units lateral to lower edge of spinous process of 3rd lumbar vertebra.	Directly on superior clunial nerve, lumbar nerve plexus (deeper), branches of lumbar artery and vein.
M-BW-25	Shi Qi Zhui Xia - Below 17th Vertebra	Back midline, 1 vertebra below GV-3, at lumbro-sacral joint (5th lumbar and 1st sacral vertebras).	Medial branch of posterior ramus of 5th lumbar nerve, accompanying arterial and venous branches.
M-BW-35	Jia Ji - Lining the Spine	48 points located at each vertebra, 0.5–1 unit lateral to midline + lower end of spinous process.	Each point supplied by a medial branch of the dorsal ramus of its corresponding spinal nerve, and accompanying artery and vein. 24 bilateral points (48 total).
M-CA-18	Zi Gong - Infant's Palace	Abdomen, 4 units below navel, 3 units lateral to CO-3 and body midline.	Iliohypogastric nerve, superficial epigastric artery and vein
M-HN-1	Si Shen Cong - Alert Spirit Quartet	Head, 4 points, 1 unit in front, behind and lateral to GV-20 (1 unit from GV-20 on all 4 sides).	Great occipital nerve, auriculotemporal nerve, lateral branches of frontal nerve, occipital artery, lateral frontal artery, superficial temporal artery.
• M-HN-3	Yin Tang - Hall of Impression	Front midline, in recess halfway between medial ends of eyebrows (glabella), also called GV-24.5.	Superior palpebral branch of supratrochlearis nerve, medial frontal artery and vein.
• M-HN-4	Shan Gen - Mountain's Base	Front midline, lowest point on bridge of nose, halfway between inner canthi of left + right eyes.	
M-HN-6	Yu Yao - Fish Waist	In recess at center of eyebrow, directly above eye pupil (when looking straight ahead).	Directly on lateral branch of frontal nerve, lateral branches of frontal artery and vein.
• M-HN-9	Tai Yang - Sun	Temple, in recess 1 unit posterior to the midpoint between outer canthus of eye and tip of eyebrow.	Auriculotemporal and facial nerves, zygomaticotemporalis nerve (deeper), venous network within the temporalis fascia, deep temporal arteries and veins.
• M-HN-14	Bi Tong - Nose Passage	Side of nose at cheek, in recess at lateral lower edge of nasal bone, at upper end of groove.	Anterior ethmoidal nerve, infratrochlearis nerve, branch of infraorbital nerve, branches of facial artery and vein.
M-HN-29	Xin Shi - New Recognition	Back of neck, 1.5 units lateral to lower edge of spinous process of 3rd cervical vertebra.	
M-HN-30	Bai Lao - Hundred Labors	Back of neck, 2 units above and 1 unit lateral to GV-14 .	Note: GV-14 is located at midline of spine, at level of shoulder, between spinous processes of 7th cervical and 1st thoracic vertebras.
M-HN-31	Chong Gu - Lofty Bone	Back of neck, below spinous process of 6th cervical vertebra.	
• M-HN-41	Jing Bi - Neck and Arm	1/3 distance from medial to lateral tip of clavicle, 1 unit up, at rear edge of sternocleidomastoid m.	Anterior branch of supraclavicular nerve, brachial plexus root (deeper), branches of superficial carotid and transverse cervical arteries and veins.
• M-LE-13	Lan Wei Xue - Appendix Orifice	Lower leg, at tender point about 2 units below ST-36, 1 unit above and slightly lateral to ST-37.	Lateral sural cutaneous nerve, deep peroneal nerve (deeper), anterior tibial artery and vein, (this point relates to loss of locomotive functions in lower extremities).
M-LE-16	Xi Yan - Eye of Knee	2 points, in recesses below kneecap, medial and lateral to patellar ligament, when knee is bent.	2 bilateral points (4 total). Inner acupoint is usually labeled M-LE-16 (Xi Yan); outer acupoint is usually labeled ST-35 (Du Bi).
• M-LE-23	Dan Nang Xue - Gallbladder Orifice	Outer lower leg, at tender point 1–2 units below GB-34.	Lateral sural cutaneous nerve, directly on peroneal nerve (deeper), (point relates to loss of locomotive functions in lower extremities).

Extra Acupoints

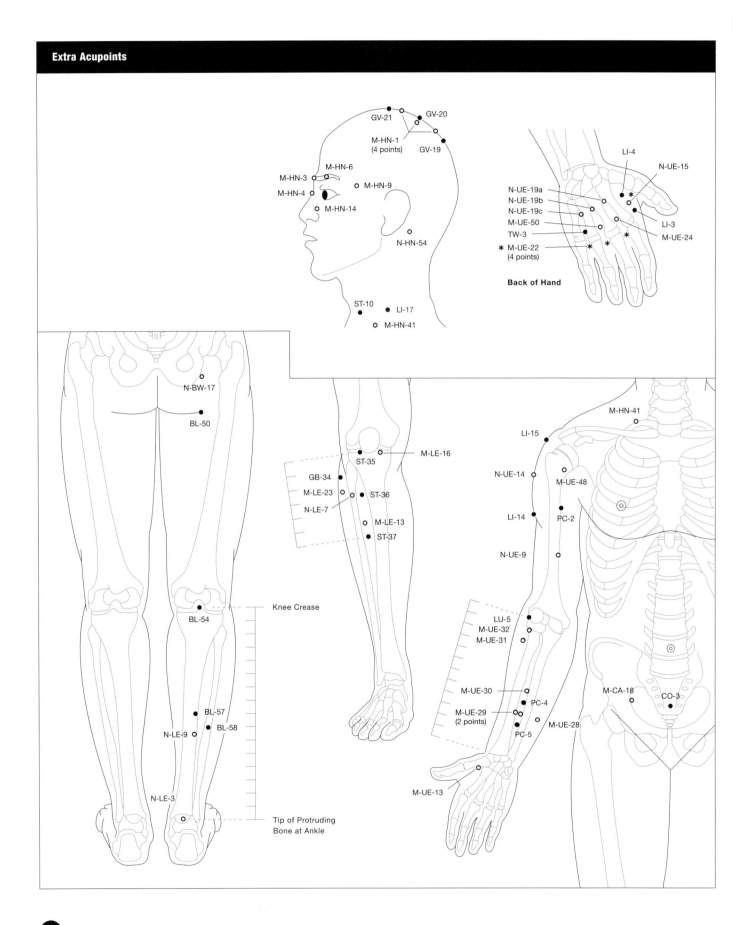

GV-21
GV-20
M-HN-1 (4 points)
GV-19
M-HN-6
M-HN-3
M-HN-4
M-HN-9
M-HN-14
N-HN-54
ST-10
LI-17
M-HN-41

LI-4
N-UE-15
N-UE-19a
N-UE-19b
N-UE-19c
M-UE-50
TW-3
LI-3
M-UE-24
* M-UE-22 (4 points)

Back of Hand

N-BW-17
BL-50

M-LE-16
ST-35
GB-34
M-LE-23
ST-36
N-LE-7
M-LE-13
ST-37

Knee Crease

BL-54

BL-57
BL-58
N-LE-9

N-LE-3

Tip of Protruding
Bone at Ankle

M-HN-41
LI-15
N-UE-14
M-UE-48
LI-14
PC-2
N-UE-9
LU-5
M-UE-32
M-UE-31
M-UE-30
PC-4
M-UE-29 (2 points)
M-UE-28
PC-5
M-CA-18
CO-3
M-UE-13

Symbol	Chinese Name	Location	Local Anatomy (Nerves and Blood Vessels)
• M-UE-13	Ban Men - Board's Door	Palm, 1 unit medial to LU-10 and thenar eminence (bulge below thumb), further into hand.	Muscular (recurrent) branch of median nerve, venules of thumb draining to cephalic vein.
• M-UE-22	Ba Xie - Eight Evils	Back of hand or clenched fist, between heads of metacarpal bones (knuckles), 4 points per hand.	Dorsal digital nerves, arteries and veins; branches of common palmar digital nerves, arteries and veins; intercapital veins.
• M-UE-24	Luo Zhen - Stiff Neck	Back of hand, between 2nd and 3rd metacarpal bones, 0.5 unit proximal to base joints of fingers.	Dorsal digital and common palmar nerves, arteries and veins; branches of deep palmar arch; deep terminal branch of ulnar nerve.
• M-UE-28	Ding Shu - Carbuncle's Hollow	Ulnar side of forearm, 4 units above ulnar end of wrist crease, between flexor muscles at ulna.	Ulnar nerve.
M-UE-29	Er Bai - Two Whites	Forearm, 4 units above middle of wrist crease, 1 point on each side of tendon (palmaris longus).	2 bilateral points (4 total). First point is beween two tendons, second point is on radial side (thumb-side) of tendons.
M-UE-30	Bi Zhong - Middle of Arm	Inner forearm, halfway between creases of wrist and elbow, between radius and ulna bones.	Directly on median nerve. Anterior and posterior interosseous nerves, median artery and vein, and interosseous arteries and veins.
• M-UE-31	Ze Xia - Below the Marsh	Thumb-side of forearm, 2 units below (distal) LU-5 and elbow crease, 1 unit below M-UE-32.	Lateral antebrachial cutaneous nerve, radial nerve, branches of radial recurrent artery and vein, cephalic vein.
• M-UE-32	Ze Qian - Before the Marsh	Thumb-side of forearm, 1 unit below (distal), and slightly medial to, LU-5 and elbow crease.	Lateral antebrachial cutaneous nerve, radial nerve, branches of radial recurrent artery and vein, cephalic vein.
M-UE-48	Jian Nei Ling - Shoulder's Inner Tomb	Halfway between end of anterior axillary crease (armpit) and LI-15 (shoulder), when arm hangs.	Posterior branch of supraclavicular nerve, axillary nerve (deeper), anterior and posterior branches of circumflex humeral artery and vein.
• M-UE-50	Shang Ba Xie - Upper Eight Evils	Back of hand,* between 3rd and 4th metacarpal bones, 0.5 unit proximal to base joints of fingers.	Dorsal digital and common palmar digital nerves, arteries and veins. (*4 points per hand, although 3 align exactly with LI-4, M-UE-24, and TW-3).
N-BW-17	Zuo Gu - Ischium Bone	Buttock, 1 unit below the midpoint between protruding bone at hip (trochanter) and tailbone.	Inferior clunial nerve, branches of inferior gluteal nerve (deeper), root of posterior cutaneous nerve of thigh (deeper), inferior gluteal artery and vein.
• N-HN-54	An Mian - Quiet Sleep	Behind ear, below occiput on posterior edge of mastoid, halfway between TW-17 and GB-20.	Minor occipital nerve, branch of great auricular nerve, occipital artery and vein.
N-LE-3	Gen Ping - Level with Heel	On Achilles tendon at back of ankle, on a line between protruding bones at both sides of ankle.	Branch of sural nerve, tibial nerve (deeper), communicating branches of posterior tibial and peroneal arteries and veins.
• N-LE-7	Li Wai - Outside the Measure	Outer lower leg below knee, 1 unit lateral to ST-36.	Lateral sural cutaneous nerve and cutaneous branch of saphenous nerve (near surface), deep peroneal nerve (deeper).
• N-LE-9	Gen Jin - Rigid Heel	Back of leg, 9.5 units below midpoint of knee crease, below BL-57 and gastrocnemius m. (calf).	Directly on sural nerve. Tibial nerve (deeper), lesser saphenous vein, posterior tibial artery and vein (deeper).
• N-UE-9	Gong Zhong - Middle of Humerus	Upper arm, in biceps and brachialis muscles, 2.5 units below PC-2, 4.5 units below axillary fold.	Medial cutaneous nerve, musculocutaneous nerve (deeper).
N-UE-14	Nao Shang - Above Scapula	Upper arm, in middle of deltoid muscle, approximately between LI-14 and LI-15.	Lateral cutaneous nerve of arm, axillary nerve (deeper), circumflex artery and vein.
N-UE-15	Hu Bian - Beside the Tiger	Back of hand in web of thumb, between LI-3 and LI-4.	Superficial branch of radial nerve.
• N-UE-19a	Yao Tong #1 - Low Back Pain #1	Back of hand, at forked recess where 2nd and 3rd metacarpal bones merge.	Similar to M-UE-24. However, this point is more painful when pressed; same location as M-UE-25 (Wei Ling).
N-UE-19b	Yao Tong #2 - Low Back Pain #2	Back of hand, at forked recess where 3rd and 4th metacarpal bones merge.	
N-UE-19c	Yao Tong #3 - Low Back Pain #3	Back of hand, at forked recess where 4th and 5th metacarpal bones merge.	

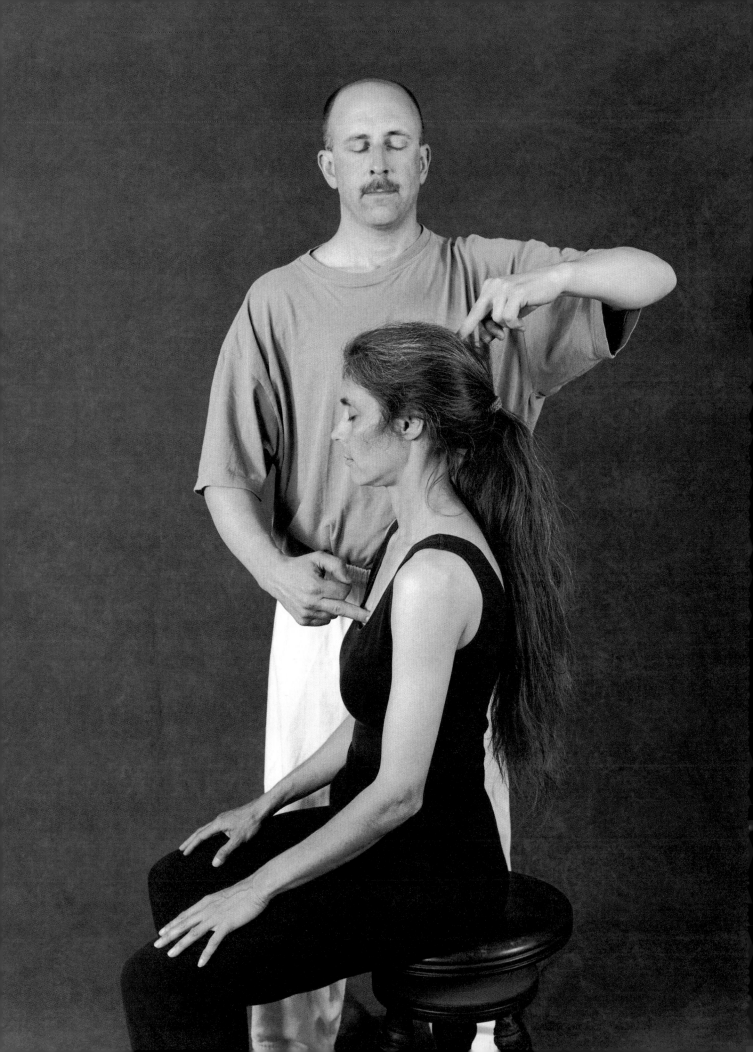

All healing traditions are concerned with the diagnosis, treatment, and prevention of illness, and the promotion of health and wellness. Naturally, the methods by which this is accomplished vary widely based on the particular healing system or procedure. For example, acupuncture (surgical), moxibustion (heat), cupping (suction), herbal medicine (dietary), massage (physical touch), meditation (mental) and physical exercise (movement) are all methods of curing illness and promoting health. Most of these methods

HEALING APPLICATIONS

are typically associated with Eastern medicine, although Western medicine has many equivalents, such as chiropractic, homeopathy, reflexology, and physical therapy. All healing arts have specific limitations, but work well when practiced within the parameters of that system. Many times different approaches are combined for great effect. The following pages briefly outline common massage and revival techniques practiced in the martial and healing arts. These skills should always be learned from qualified instructors.

Massage is essentially the art of healing by touch—rubbing, pressing, sliding, tapping, slapping, kneading and shaking. Many different massage techniques and systems have evolved over a period of thousands of years as a part of the natural healing systems of many different cultures, both Eastern and Western. Today, many different forms of massage exist, which are used to provide a wide variety of benefits, including stress reduction, pain relief, muscle therapy, mental and emotional balancing, and acceleration of the body's natural healing processes.

Types of Massage

Generally speaking, there are three basic types of massage treatment: body massage, acupoint massage, and nerve-ending massage. In many Eastern medical practices, these different approaches are integrated into comprehensive systems, intimately linked to meridian/acupoint theory. Western systems tend to be based on anatomy and physiology.

Body Massage

Body massage involves manipulation of muscles, joints and various tissues. It can involve a range of actions, such as rubbing, pressing, pushing, pulling, tapping, slapping, kneading, shaking and vibrating. This type of massage increases the flow of blood into the area being worked, helps remove accumulated acids and toxins, and assists in the elimination of stagnant Qi. Body massage is often used to relieve pain or soreness, relax tense muscles, reduce bruises, or accelerate the healing of injuries. In some practices, this type of massage is also used to stimulate the nervous, skeletal or lymphatic systems, or to invigorate a person who is chronically tired or weak. Swedish Massage is a system of body massage familiar to Westerners.

Acupoint Massage

Acupoint massage involves stimulating specific acupoints and meridians to manipulate one's Qi-flow. This is done to restore the body's natural energetic balance and assist its ability to heal itself from a wide range of disharmonies or illnesses. Acupoint massage is based on the same principles as acupuncture, but stimulates the points by using one's fingers (also hands, knuckles, elbows and feet), rather than inserting needles into the body. While acupoints affected by finger pressure are far less than those affected by needling, massage has the benefit of being noninvasive. Thus, it can be practiced by anyone without undergoing intensive medical training and licensing.

Chinese Acupressure and Japanese Shiatsu are common systems incorporating this type of massage. Acupressure tends to focus more on acupoint manipulation and less so on meridians, whereas Shiatsu tends to emphasize meridians and uses stronger, rhythmic pressure. Western medicine also uses pressure point techniques, although, they are described in neurological terms and focus primarily on treating neuromuscular problems.

Nerve-Ending Massage

This form of massage involves rubbing or pressing the endings of nerves and meridians, which are mostly located on the hands, feet and ears. Each of these body parts is thought to be a microcosm of the entire body, and each is divided into zones that correspond to specific regions. Zones are selected and massaged based on the specific disharmony or illness to be treated. *Reflexology*, which developed in Europe and America during the 19th century, is a well known form of nerve-ending massage that may have evolved from older Chinese systems. The scientific basis for nerve-ending massage is not known, but may coincide with Western medicine's identification of more than 7000 nerve endings in the foot that connect with the spinal cord and brain to all areas of the body.

Types of Massage

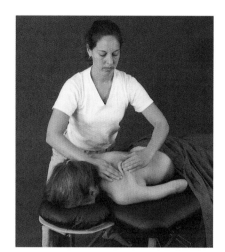

Body Massage

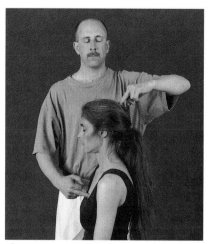

Acupoint Massage

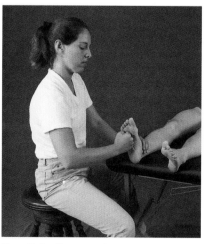

Nerve-Ending Massage

Simple Acupressure

Like most healing arts, massage is a vast and complex subject, well beyond the scope of this book. However, there are some simple acupressure techniques that are easily learned, which can be applied to one's self or another person, either to alleviate simple health problems or to maintain a balanced energetic state. Thirteen typical self-applied techniques are outlined on the following pages. They should be thought of as first-aid or preventive procedures; not as a solution for more serious health conditions that require the attention of expert medical professionals.

Basic Principles

The following basic principles generally apply to most acupressure massage techniques:

1. Make sure you are calm, relaxed, and your mind is focused on what you are trying to accomplish. A few minutes of meditation, deep breathing and/or a quick mini-massage (rub your entire body from head to toe) can help quiet the mind and relax your muscles.

2. Throughout the acupressure procedure, you should breathe slowly and deeply down into the abdomen, expanding it as you inhale and contracting it as you exhale. Deep breathing increases the circulation of blood and Qi, elevates oxygen intake, promotes relaxation and helps keep the mind focused. This form of breathing should be practiced by both the masseuse and the patient.

3. Accurately locate the acupoint, otherwise acupressure massage is relatively ineffectual. If you are off by a half inch, the acupoint may be unaffected.

4. Your minds intent is an important part of the acupressure process. Try to concentrate on, and visualize, the process you are attempting to accomplish. If you are trying to stimulate the flow of energy into an area to relieve a muscle spasm, visualize this process occurring. Daydreaming while pressing an acupoint can be very counterproductive.

5. If you are working on another person, keep both of your hands on the patient at all times, even if you are only pressing an acupoint with one hand. This helps maintain a continuous energy-flow between the healer and patient.

6. When massaging bilateral acupoints, work both sides of the body for the same amount of time. You may either press both acupoints at the same time, or one after the other.

7. Apply pressure using your fingertips, thumb, or your entire hand, as shown on later pages. Apply pressure gradually for the first 5 to 10 seconds, maintain pressure for 1 to 3 minutes, then release pressure gradually for the last 5 to 10 seconds. Pressure should be firm, but not painful. Sensitive or bony parts of the body (e.g., the face) usually require less pressure, whereas the back and chest require more. Generally, about 15 pounds per square inch is the maximum amount of pressure that should be applied. You can use a bathroom scale to learn what this feels like.

8. When you are finished, gently shake your hands several times, breathe deeply, and relax for a few minutes before continuing on to other activities.

Precautions

When applying acupressure techniques, observe the following precautions: Do not massage lesions, sores, lumps, tumors, open wounds or burns. Do not use massage on persons with cardiovascular or liver problems, serious medical issues, infectious diseases, or psychological disorders. Do not massage pregnant women unless you are a qualified professional, as certain acupoints can trigger a miscarriage if improperly stimulated.

Methods for Stimulating Acupoints

There are many different methods for stimulating acupoints. When comparing various massage systems, it is not uncommon to note contradictory theories and stimulation methods. Nonetheless, most work when practiced within the context of that healing art. One typical approach, which can be used with the techniques on the following pages, is based on applying one of three forms of pressure to stimulate the acupoints: strengthening, dispersing and calming. All of these methods seek to restore the body's natural energetic balance, and strengthen Qi-flow. The stimulation method used is based on the disharmony to be treated, and the quality of one's Qi.

Tonifying Pressure

This is used to strengthen weak Qi. Apply stationary pressure to the acupoint for 1 to 3 minutes. Usually your finger or thumb presses perpendicular to the acupoint.

Dispersing Pressure

This is used to disperse stagnant or blocked Qi. Apply moving pressure to the acupoint for 1 to 3 minutes. Two common methods of applying dispersing pressure are: 1) apply firm pressure to the acupoint, then rotate your finger in a circular motion, alternating between clockwise and counterclockwise directions; or 2) alternately press in and release out of the acupoint, using a "pumping" action.

Calming Pressure

This is used to calm overactive Qi. Two common methods of applying pressure are: 1) lightly cover the point with your palm, or 2) lightly rub or stroke the area with your thumb, finger(s) or palm for 1 to 3 minutes.

Other Approaches

Some massage systems focus on the degree of stimulation (strong, moderate, light), rather than the specific finger actions just outlined. Other systems focus more on creating an energetic connection, and less so on finger skills or the degree of stimulation. Some healing arts merely apply steady, penetrating pressure in virtually all situations.

1. Headache Release

LI-4, GB-20, M-HN-9, GB-13, ST-8

Disperse LI-4, which is in the web of the thumb (center of muscle), pressing slightly toward the index finger (do not press this acupoint during pregnancy). Disperse both GB-20 acupoints (neck) as outlined in technique 3. Disperse both M-HN-9 points on the temple, using a circular action that reverses every 30 seconds. Disperse GB-13, then ST-8. For stress related or lateral headaches, disperse GB-41 (foot) and TW-5 (wrist), For frontal headaches, disperse GV-23 (forehead) and LV-3 (foot), and tonify ST-36.

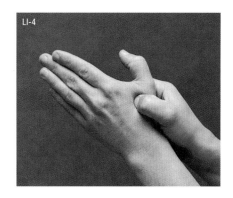

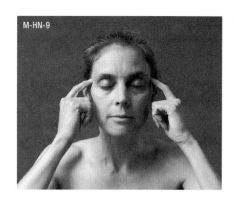

2. Mind Harmonizer

M-HN-3 + GV-20, ST-36

Gently disperse M-HN-3 (between the eyebrows), as you disperse GV-20 (vertex) with your palm or fingers. Then tonify both ST-36 acupoints on the outer knee. These three points improve general brain functions and have a calming, centering effect. They also help headaches. To improve concentration, additionally tonify SP-3 (foot) and ST-40 (lower leg). To improve memory, tonify KI-3, BL-23 and BL-20. To boost immune functions, tonify SP-6, ST-36 and LI-10. To energize the mind and body, tonify GV-4, CO-4, SP-6 and ST-36.

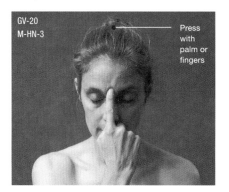

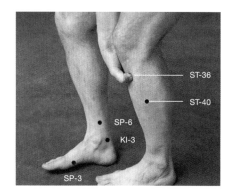

3. Neck Release

SI-12, GB-21, GB-20, LI-4, M-UE-24

These acupoints can be used to reduce tension or pain. Disperse SI-12, just above the spine of the scapula, using the weight of your hanging arm to apply finger pressure. Use the same technique to disperse GB-21, which is on the muscle at the top of the shoulder, halfway between the C7 vertebra and the protruding bone at the top of the shoulder. Disperse both GB-20 points at the base of the skull with your thumbs. Additionally, tonifying LI-4 or M-UE-24 (back of hand) may also help. Points listed under "Shoulder Release" also work.

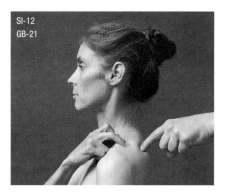

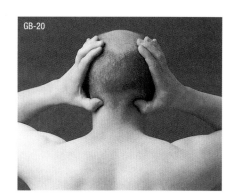

4. Shoulder Release

TW-14 + LI-15, SI-11

These acupoints can be used to reduce tension or pain. Disperse TW-14 and LI-15. You can press both points at the same time using your thumb and index finger; or one point first, then the other. These points are next to each other, and are located by raising your arm to the side and feeling for the two depressions on each side of the tendon. Dispersing SI-11 with your finger is difficult, as it is located in the center of the scapula. However, you can self-massage this point by lying on a golf or tennis ball, or by leaning into the corner of a chair.

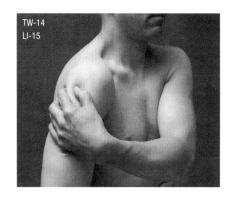

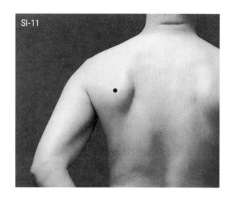

All techniques shown can be applied to one's self or others. These treatments can be used to reduce pain and muscle tension, accelerate healing, or optimize health.

Caution:
Do not press LI-4, GB-21, SP-6, SP-9 and BL-60 during pregnancy; or GV-20 on persons with high blood pressure.

5. Abdominal Release

PC-6, CO-12 + LV-13, ST-25, ST-36, SP-4

These acupoints can be used to reduce simple indigestion or nausea, such as motion sickness. Disperse or calm PC-6 with your thumb (middle of the inner arm, two thumb-widths above the wrist crease). Disperse CO-12 with your middle finger or palm (four thumb-widths above the navel), as you disperse LV-13 with your thumb (below 11th rib). Also disperse ST-25 (two thumb-widths lateral to navel), ST-36 (four finger-widths below lower-outer corner of kneecap, where muscle moves when foot is flexed) and SP-4 (foot).

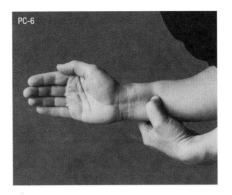

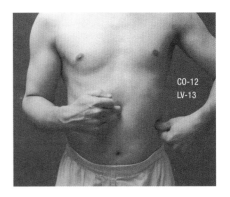

6. Elbow Release

LI-11, TW-5, TW-10, LI-4

These acupoints can be used to reduce tension or pain, and are also useful for shoulder problems. Disperse LI-11 with your thumb. This point is located on the outer elbow, at the end of the elbow crease. Disperse TW-5 with your thumb. This point is located on the outer arm, two thumb-widths above the wrist, between the ulna and radius bones. Additionally, you can also disperse TW-10 (one thumb-width above point of elbow) and LI-4 (web of thumb, see technique 1), and tonify GB-34 (see technique 10).

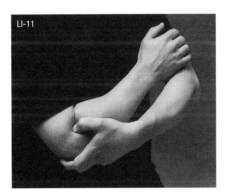

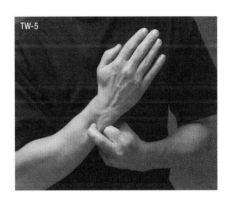

7. Wrist Release

LI-5 + SI-5, TW-4

These acupoints can be used to reduce tension or pain. Firmly disperse LI-5 and SI-5 at the same time, using your thumb and middle fingers. These points are in the depressions at the end of the wrist crease. Disperse TW-4 with your thumb. This point is located in a recess just lateral to the middle of the wrist crease, on the back of the wrist. The acupoints listed under "Elbow Release" are also helpful. For carpal tunnel syndrome, disperse PC-7 (middle of the wrist crease) and PC-6 (two thumb-widths above the wrist crease).

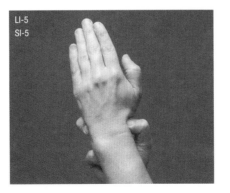

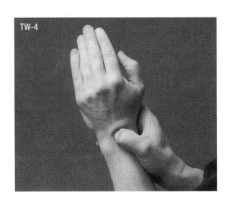

8. Hand Release

LI-4 + SI-3, M-UE-22

These acupoints can be used to reduce stiffness and pain, and are often utilized with the previous "Wrist Release" acupoints. Disperse LI-4 with your thumb, as you press SI-3 with your middle finger. The SI-3 acupoint is located on the edge of the hand, in the recess above the knuckle of the little finger (proximal to the joint). For finger pain or numbness, disperse one or more of three acupoints, all called M-UE-22. These acupoints are located between the base joints of the fingers. You can also disperse TW-5 (see technique 6).

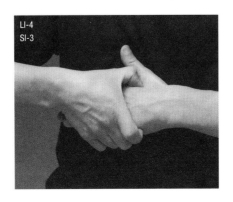

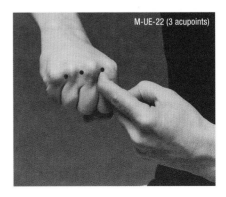

9. Back Release

BL-23, GB-30

These acupoints can be used to reduce tension, numbness, or lower back pain. Firmly disperse both BL-23 acupoints with your thumbs, or recline on top of two tennis balls. These points are located two finger-widths lateral to the midline of the spine, about level with the navel. Firmly disperse both GB-30 acupoints, using your thumb or fists; or you can also recline on top of your fists. These points are located on the buttocks in the hip joint, one third the distance from the protruding bone at hip to the tailbone. Some healers disperse GB-30 and BL-26, and tonify BL-23.

Distant Acupoints: Points on the hand and leg can also reduce back pain. Strongly tonify LI-4 (see technique 1), then two adjacent points, N-UE-15 and an "extra point" (when using these two points, press the hand opposite the side with pain). Next, strongly tonify N-UE-19a and N-UE-19c, while bending and rotating your back. For lower back pain, dispersing BL-54 (knee) and BL-60 (outer ankle) also helps (some healers tonify). For pain along the spine, stimulate GV-26 (center of upper lip) using your fingernail, and SI-3 on the hand (see technique 8), followed by BL-62 in the recess below the protruding outer anklebone.

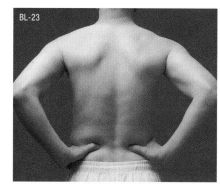

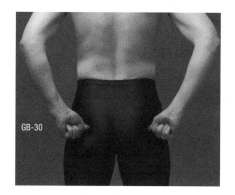

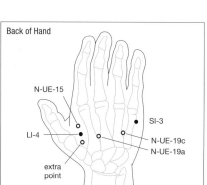

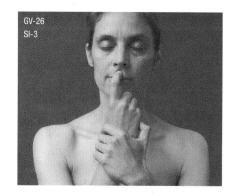

10. Hip Release

GB-30, GB-29, GB-34, LI-4

These acupoints can be used to reduce tension or pain. Disperse both GB-30 acupoints in the hip joint, as described in the previous "Back Release." Disperse both GB-29 acupoints with your thumbs. These points are located halfway between the front upper-edge of the hipbone and the protruding bone at the side of the hip. Tonify GB-34 at the outer lower leg. This point is located about one inch below the knee, in the recess anterior and below the head of the fibula. Tonify LI-4 in the web of the thumb, as described in technique 1.

11. Leg Release

GB-31, GB-34, BL-50; ST-36, GB-34, BL-57

For thigh pain, disperse GB-31 with your thumb. This point is on the outer side of the thigh, at the end of the middle finger when your arm hangs at your side. Then disperse GB-34 at the outer lower leg (see technique 10). Disperse BL-50 with your middle finger, or recline on your fist. This point is on the back of the leg, in the center of the crease below the buttock. For aching, tired legs, tonify ST-36 and GB-34, and disperse BL-57 (base of calf muscle in "v"). ST-36 is below the outer knee, where the muscle moves when the foot is flexed.

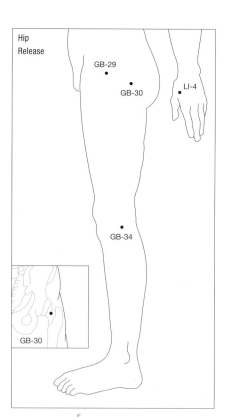

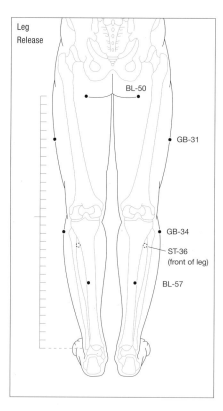

12. Knee Release

ST-35 + M-LE-16, BL-54, GB-34, SP-9 + ST-36
These acupoints can be used to reduce stiffness
or pain. Disperse ST-35 and M-LE-16, which are
located in the recesses below the inner and outer
corners of the kneecap. Disperse BL-54, which is in
the center of the back of the knee. Disperse GB-34
at the lower outer leg, as described in technique 10
(this point increases circulation). Disperse ST-36
(outer knee) and SP-9 (in recess at inner side of
knee, below the protruding tibia). Disperse SP-10
and ST-34, which are located above the knee.

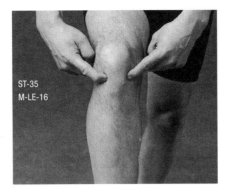

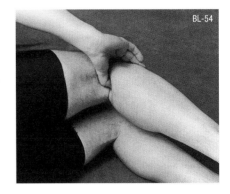

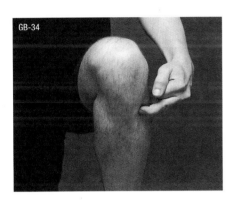

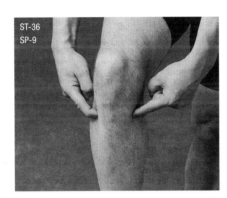

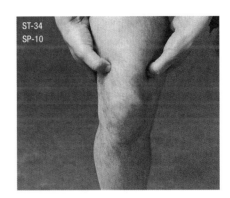

13. Ankle/Foot Release

KI-3, BL-60, ST-41, SP-6, GB-39, BL-57
These points can be used to reduce tension and pain.
Disperse KI-3 and BL-60, which are on opposite sides
of the ankle, in the recess between the anklebone
and Achilles tendon. You can press these points at
the same time or singly. Disperse ST-41, which is
between the tendons of the big toe and toes, level
with the outer anklebone. For injuries to the ligaments
on the inner side, disperse SP-6; for the outer side,
disperse GB-39. Tonifying GB-34 can also be helpful.
For pain in the sole, disperse BL-57, KI-3 and BL-60.

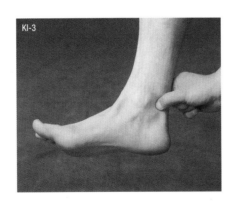

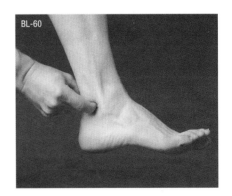

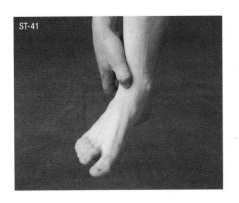

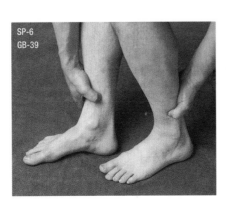

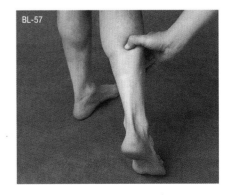

HEALING ACUPOINTS

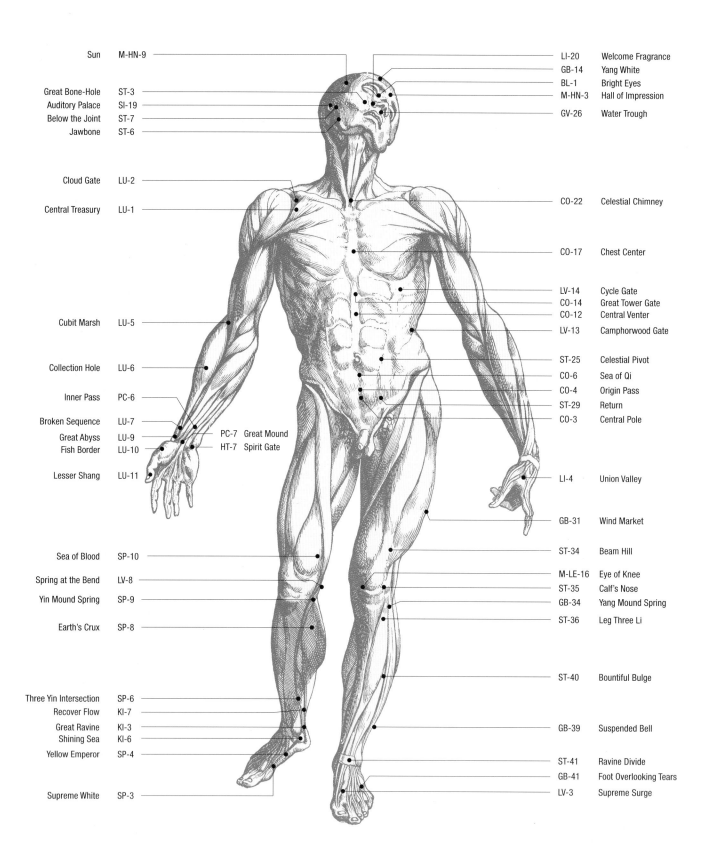

Sun — M-HN-9

Great Bone-Hole — ST-3
Auditory Palace — SI-19
Below the Joint — ST-7
Jawbone — ST-6

Cloud Gate — LU-2

Central Treasury — LU-1

Cubit Marsh — LU-5

Collection Hole — LU-6

Inner Pass — PC-6

Broken Sequence — LU-7
Great Abyss — LU-9
Fish Border — LU-10

Lesser Shang — LU-11

Sea of Blood — SP-10
Spring at the Bend — LV-8
Yin Mound Spring — SP-9
Earth's Crux — SP-8

Three Yin Intersection — SP-6
Recover Flow — KI-7
Great Ravine — KI-3
Shining Sea — KI-6
Yellow Emperor — SP-4

Supreme White — SP-3

PC-7 — Great Mound
HT-7 — Spirit Gate

LI-20 — Welcome Fragrance
GB-14 — Yang White
BL-1 — Bright Eyes
M-HN-3 — Hall of Impression
GV-26 — Water Trough

CO-22 — Celestial Chimney

CO-17 — Chest Center

LV-14 — Cycle Gate
CO-14 — Great Tower Gate
CO-12 — Central Venter
LV-13 — Camphorwood Gate

ST-25 — Celestial Pivot
CO-6 — Sea of Qi
CO-4 — Origin Pass
ST-29 — Return
CO-3 — Central Pole

LI-4 — Union Valley

GB-31 — Wind Market

ST-34 — Beam Hill
M-LE-16 — Eye of Knee
ST-35 — Calf's Nose
GB-34 — Yang Mound Spring
ST-36 — Leg Three Li

ST-40 — Bountiful Bulge

GB-39 — Suspended Bell

ST-41 — Ravine Divide
GB-41 — Foot Overlooking Tears
LV-3 — Supreme Surge

120

The illustrations on these pages show 100 common acupoints used in Eastern healing arts, such as massage and acupuncture. Each acupoint is labeled using both its alphanumeric symbol, and the English translation of the acupoint's Chinese name. Korean and Japanese translations are usually similar, if not identical. Detailed drawings and anatomical descriptions of acupoints are contained in the *Eastern Concepts* chapter.

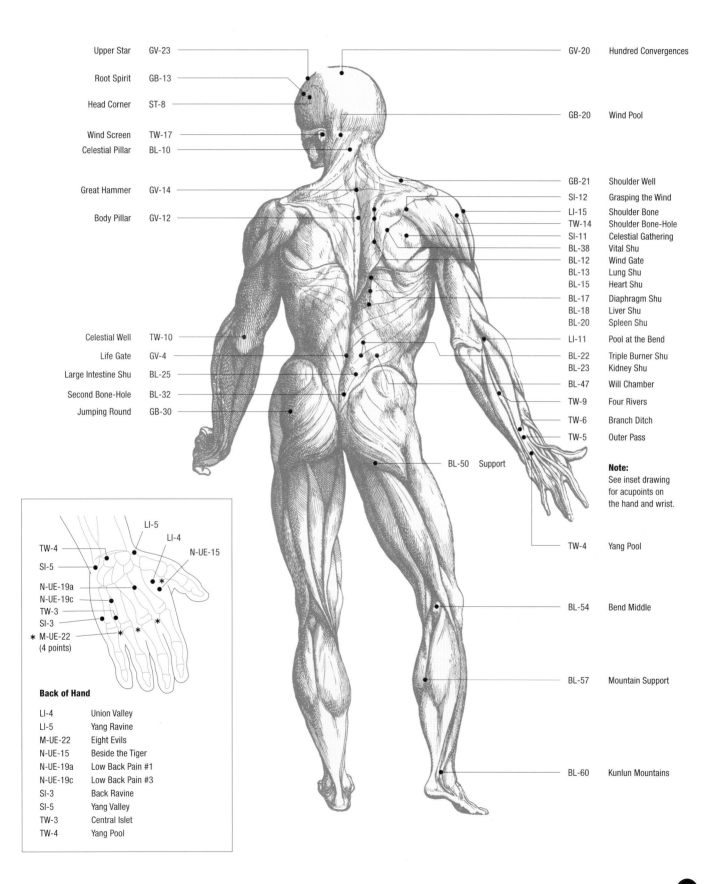

Upper Star	GV-23
Root Spirit	GB-13
Head Corner	ST-8
Wind Screen	TW-17
Celestial Pillar	BL-10
Great Hammer	GV-14
Body Pillar	GV-12
Celestial Well	TW-10
Life Gate	GV-4
Large Intestine Shu	BL-25
Second Bone-Hole	BL-32
Jumping Round	GB-30

GV-20	Hundred Convergences
GB-20	Wind Pool
GB-21	Shoulder Well
SI-12	Grasping the Wind
LI-15	Shoulder Bone
TW-14	Shoulder Bone-Hole
SI-11	Celestial Gathering
BL-38	Vital Shu
BL-12	Wind Gate
BL-13	Lung Shu
BL-15	Heart Shu
BL-17	Diaphragm Shu
BL-18	Liver Shu
BL-20	Spleen Shu
LI-11	Pool at the Bend
BL-22	Triple Burner Shu
BL-23	Kidney Shu
BL-47	Will Chamber
TW-9	Four Rivers
TW-6	Branch Ditch
TW-5	Outer Pass

Note:
See inset drawing for acupoints on the hand and wrist.

TW-4	Yang Pool
BL-54	Bend Middle
BL-57	Mountain Support
BL-60	Kunlun Mountains

BL-50   Support

Back of Hand

LI-4	Union Valley
LI-5	Yang Ravine
M-UE-22	Eight Evils
N-UE-15	Beside the Tiger
N-UE-19a	Low Back Pain #1
N-UE-19c	Low Back Pain #3
SI-3	Back Ravine
SI-5	Yang Valley
TW-3	Central Islet
TW-4	Yang Pool

LI-5
LI-4
TW-4
SI-5
N-UE-15
N-UE-19a
N-UE-19c
TW-3
SI-3
★ M-UE-22
(4 points)

REVIVAL TECHNIQUES

Overview

It is not uncommon for breathing or heart functions to cease when a person is rendered unconscious. This may result from a choke hold cutting off the air or blood supply, or by striking certain acupoints or vital targets. Restoration of breathing and heart functions is often quite simple for someone with proper medical training. For someone without training, or in the absence of immediate attention, an individual might easily die or suffer permanent brain damage.

In the martial arts, Eastern revival methods are often used to revive a person who is dazed or unconscious. Many of these methods evolved during prior centuries, and were secretly studied along with pressure point strikes. During the twentieth century, many of these secret methods gradually became known to the general public.

Today, numerous revival methods exist. This chapter will present those most typically used in the martial arts. These procedures should be learned from a qualified practitioner. They are considered to be "first aid," and are not a substitute for qualified medical attention. In any medical emergency, always seek the aid of qualified medical personnel. Never attempt to move anyone if you suspect serious injuries; you may do more harm than good, and be legally liable.

Legal Concerns

Use of accepted Eastern revival techniques in the United States, which are well established and proven in Asia, may leave you vulnerable to a lawsuit, since they are not currently approved by the American Medical Association. Cardiopulmonary Resuscitation (CPR) and other Western first aid procedures are easily learned and often taught for free at the community level. Incorrect application of Eastern or Western revival techniques may leave you legally responsible for your actions. The material presented in this section is neither an endorsement of, nor a guarantee that any of these techniques will be safe or effective in any medical emergency.

Revival Techniques

The following revival techniques are those most commonly used, and are easily learned. Many others exist, including some that rely on precise pressure point knowledge and/or Qi manipulation. Before applying any revival technique, check the patient's air passage to make sure it is clear. Food, water, a foreign object or the tongue can cause a blockage, which must be addressed. Loss of consciousness may be accompanied by cyanosis (bluish or purplish discoloration of skin due to lack of oxygen) or incontinence (inability to control waste functions). Do not attempt to move anyone if you suspect serious injuries (e.g., spinal fracture).

1. Knee-to-Spine Revival

This is used to restore breathing functions or revive a person who has fainted. Maneuver the patient into a sitting position with one leg crossed. Support the head and avoid sharp movements, or you may cause whiplash. Stand behind the patient with your knee pressing into the spine, between the shoulder blades. Spread your fingers and place your hands on the lower chest. Pull back the chest and shoulders as you press your knee forward into the spine. This action draws air into the lungs. When the ribs are open as far as they will go, release them, returning to the starting position. This action expels air from the lungs. This inhalation-exhalation process should be repeated slowly and regularly at a rate of 4 to 6 seconds per cycle (10 to 15 times per minute), until the patient begins breathing without assistance. Your movements should encourage the natural breathing process by opening and closing the diaphragm.

2. Spine-Slap Revival

This is used to restore breathing or revive a person who has fainted. Maneuver the patient into a sitting position, with the legs extended and the hands hanging at the side. Support the head and avoid sharp movements, to avoid whiplash. Kneel to one side of the patient. Support the upper body with your left arm. Form a Palm Hand, placing your middle finger on or near the protruding bone at the base of the neck. Using the lower portion of your palm, hit firmly into the 6th and 7th thoracic vertebras, between the shoulders. This provides a shock that will often initiate breathing. Do not hit so hard as to damage vertebras or cause whiplash. This is a very old technique, but one that works well.

3. Acupoint Revival

When hitting nerves or acupoints, you may cause someone to faint. If a person is already nervous, fatigued, weak or hungry, they will be more susceptible. To revive a person who has fainted, press hard with your fingernail at: GV-26 on the upper lip (see 3.1); LI-4 at the back of the hand, in the web of the thumb (see 3.2); or KI-1 on the sole of the foot (see 3.3). Many other acupoint manipulations are used to treat injuries to specific areas of the body. Most require proper medical training.

4. Testicle Revival (lifting and dropping)

This procedure is used to treat a patient whose testicles have been kicked up into his pelvis. It is not used to restore breathing. Place the patient in a sitting position and stand behind him. Wrap your arms under the armpits and clasp your hands together (see 4A). Lift him upward a few inches and let him drop (see 4B–4C), repeating as necessary (usually 6 to 7 times). This jarring motion may cause the testicles to drop back to their original position. Seek qualified medical attention as soon as possible.

5. Testicle Revival (kicking to sacrum)

This procedure is used to treat a patient whose testicles have been kicked up into his pelvis. It is not used to restore breathing. Place the patient in a sitting position and stand behind him. Lightly kick the sacrum in the center of the hips, with the ball or sole of your foot. This may cause the testicles to drop back to their original position. Do not kick too forcefully or you may damage the sacral spine. Two methods of supporting the upper body are shown. In the first method, place your hands on the patients shoulders (see 5A). In the second method, lift one armpit, slightly elevating one buttock (see 5B).

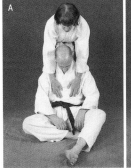 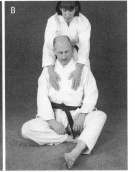 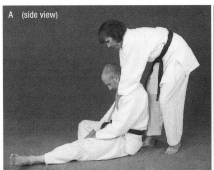 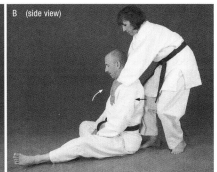

1. Knee-to-Spine Revival

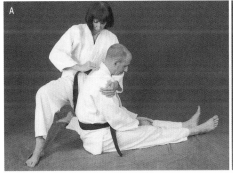 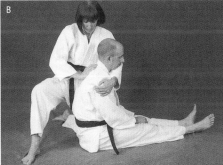 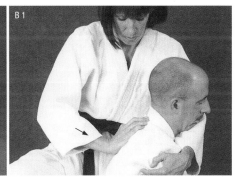

2. Spine-Slap Revival

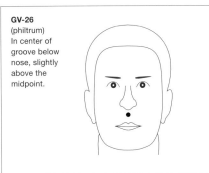

GV-26
(philtrum)
In center of
groove below
nose, slightly
above the
midpoint.

3.1 Acupoint Revival (press GV-26)

LI-4
(backhand)
Center of muscle
in web of thumb,
slightly toward
2nd metacarpal.
Do not press
if pregnant.

3.2 Acupoint Revival (press LI-4)

KI-1
(sole of foot)
In recess 1/3
the distance
from from base
of toes to heel.

3.3 Acupoint Revival (press KI-1)

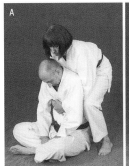 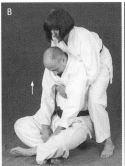 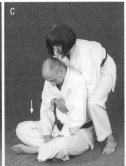

4. Testicle Revival (lifting and dropping)

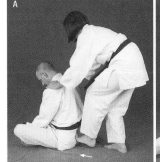 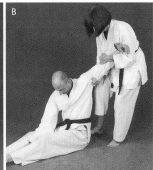

5. Testicle Revival (kicking to sacrum)

123

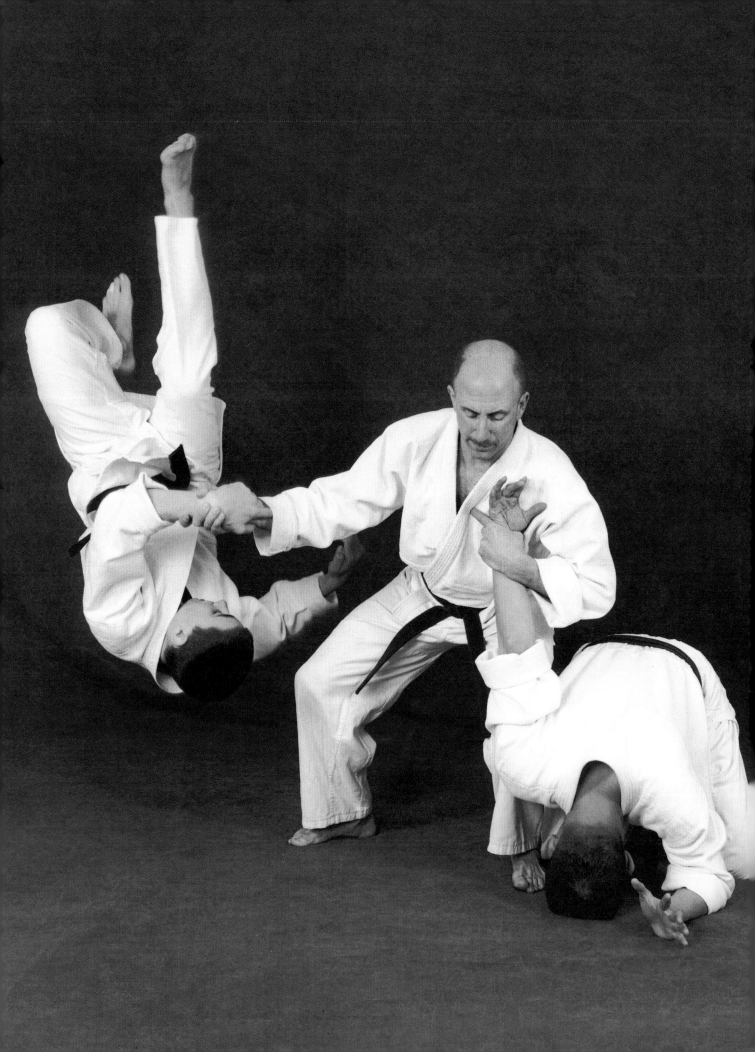

Martial artists study the human body for two purposes: to hurt and to heal. This chapter will show how Western and Eastern anatomical principles are applied to combat and self-defense. When using this knowledge it is vital to remember: the use of force to resolve a situation carries with it a social and moral responsibility to apply force in an appropriate and sensible manner. When we attempt to control another person by striking, holding or throwing, our understanding of the human body allows us not only to attack

MARTIAL APPLICATIONS

with increased efficiency, but with greater compassion. By manipulating the body's weak points, it becomes possible to immobilize an attacker without causing serious injury. To seriously injure or kill someone is not difficult. It requires no special knowledge, and often occurs unintentionally. For the skilled martial artist, the excessive use of force is an inexcusable and morally reprehensible act, deserving condemnation. One should always respect life. It is a precious gift that can never be returned once it has been taken.

ANATOMICAL TARGETS

The following drawings identify vital targets using basic Western medical terminology. Damage to these anatomically weak points can cause trauma to blood vessels, nerves, bones, tissue and joints—either separately or in unison. For example, striking the temple may cause a concussion, a skull fracture, neck trauma (whiplash), damage to cranial nerves, arteries and veins; all of the above; or none of the above (the strike could be ineffective). The level of damage depends on force, angle of attack, method of attack (strike, press, hold), hitting surface (fist, weapon), and individual anatomy (bone mass, musculature, etc.).

Head Area

The head, face and lower edge of the jaw contain numerous *cranial nerves,* well exposed to strikes or pressing holds. Head blows may cause a concussion by slamming the brain against the skull cavity (usually 180° opposite of the blow). This causes bleeding into the brain and death of brain cells, resulting in dizziness, confusion, loss of consciousness or even death. Blows to the chin are usually directed sideways causing the TMJ (joint) to fracture at the back of the mandible, especially when the jaw is open. The nose is structurally weakest when struck from the side, although a frontal blow is also painful. Eye strikes can result in corneal abrasion, globe rupture, retinal detachment or fracture of the socket surrounding the eye.

Neck Area

Major blood vessels (carotid, jugular) and nerves (cervical, supraclavicular, auricular, vagus, accessory) are all concentrated close to the sternocleidomastoid muscle, at the side of the neck. Chokes applied at this point restrict blood flow to the brain, resulting in loss of consciousness or death. Blows to the back or side of the neck can dislocate cervical vertebrae or damage nerve roots, impairing motor functions. Accessory nerve damage paralyzes sternocleidomastoid and trapezius muscles, resulting in an inability to raise the shoulder or turn the head. Violently twisting the head can fracture vertebrae, causing paralysis or death. A blow to the larynx, trachea or surrounding cartilage can cause obstruction of the airway and bleeding into the throat—injuries which can be fatal.

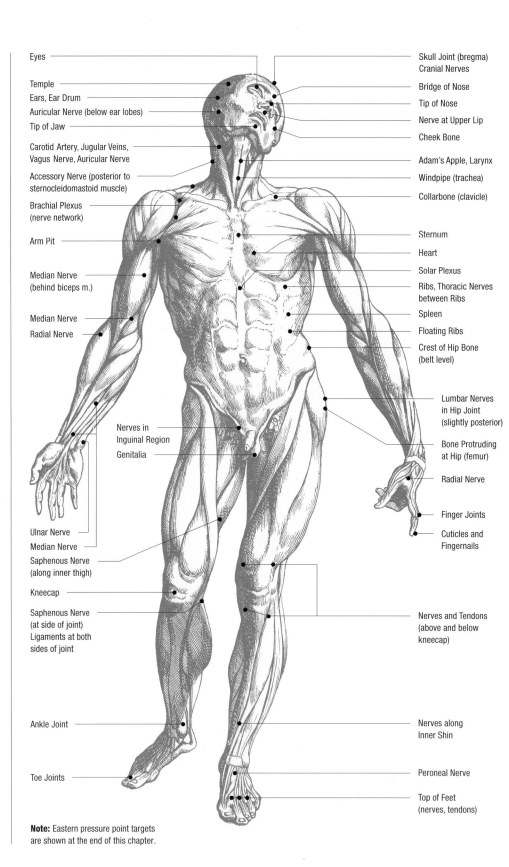

Eyes

Temple

Ears, Ear Drum

Auricular Nerve (below ear lobes)

Tip of Jaw

Carotid Artery, Jugular Veins, Vagus Nerve, Auricular Nerve

Accessory Nerve (posterior to sternocleidomastoid muscle)

Brachial Plexus (nerve network)

Arm Pit

Median Nerve (behind biceps m.)

Median Nerve

Radial Nerve

Nerves in Inguinal Region

Genitalia

Ulnar Nerve

Median Nerve

Saphenous Nerve (along inner thigh)

Kneecap

Saphenous Nerve (at side of joint) Ligaments at both sides of joint

Ankle Joint

Toe Joints

Skull Joint (bregma) Cranial Nerves

Bridge of Nose

Tip of Nose

Nerve at Upper Lip

Cheek Bone

Adam's Apple, Larynx

Windpipe (trachea)

Collarbone (clavicle)

Sternum

Heart

Solar Plexus

Ribs, Thoracic Nerves between Ribs

Spleen

Floating Ribs

Crest of Hip Bone (belt level)

Lumbar Nerves in Hip Joint (slightly posterior)

Bone Protruding at Hip (femur)

Radial Nerve

Finger Joints

Cuticles and Fingernails

Nerves and Tendons (above and below kneecap)

Nerves along Inner Shin

Peroneal Nerve

Top of Feet (nerves, tendons)

Note: Eastern pressure point targets are shown at the end of this chapter.

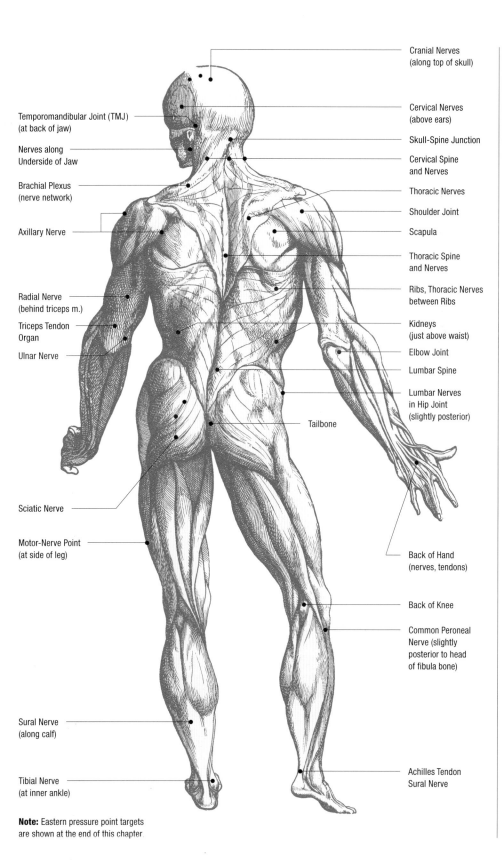

Cranial Nerves
(along top of skull)

Temporomandibular Joint (TMJ)
(at back of jaw)

Cervical Nerves
(above ears)

Nerves along
Underside of Jaw

Skull-Spine Junction

Cervical Spine
and Nerves

Brachial Plexus
(nerve network)

Thoracic Nerves

Shoulder Joint

Axillary Nerve

Scapula

Thoracic Spine
and Nerves

Radial Nerve
(behind triceps m.)

Ribs, Thoracic Nerves
between Ribs

Triceps Tendon
Organ

Kidneys
(just above waist)

Ulnar Nerve

Elbow Joint

Lumbar Spine

Lumbar Nerves
in Hip Joint
(slightly posterior)

Tailbone

Sciatic Nerve

Back of Hand
(nerves, tendons)

Motor-Nerve Point
(at side of leg)

Back of Knee

Common Peroneal
Nerve (slightly
posterior to head
of fibula bone)

Sural Nerve
(along calf)

Tibial Nerve
(at inner ankle)

Achilles Tendon
Sural Nerve

Note: Eastern pressure point targets
are shown at the end of this chapter.

Shoulder Area

The *brachial plexus* is a network of cervical and thoracic nerves (median, radial, ulnar, axillary, musculocutaneous) which form the entire nerve supply for the upper extremities and shoulder area. The nerves lie close together as they pass from the top of the shoulder, behind the collarbone, along the front of the joint, and down to the armpit, where they branch into the arm. They are very vulnerable to blows or pressure directed to the areas indicated. The collarbone is easily fractured or separated by a direct blow or fall. Joint-lock holds or a throw can dislocate the shoulder. Blows to the back of the shoulder or scapula can damage a variety of thoracic nerves (especially if near the spine).

Trunk Area

The *solar plexus* is a nerve network found below the sternum. Blows to the solar plexus hinder breathing by causing transient paralysis of the diaphragm (see *Note* on page 18). Blows to the sternum can cause trauma to the heart. Ribs are easily fractured by forceful blows (especially floating ribs) and may puncture the lungs or other organs. Lateral or posterior blows can rupture the spleen, while posterior blows to the kidneys can cause bruising or severe internal bleeding. Strikes to the genitalia are painful, but not always debilitating. Strikes to the spinal column can damage nerves, resulting in transient or permanent paralysis.

Arm and Leg Areas

The elbow, wrist and finger joints are frequently attacked with twisting or breaking holds due to their inherent weakness and susceptibility to pain. Nerve attacks to hands, fingernails and elbows are usually used to release a hold, distract, or assist applying a hold. The knee is probably the most vulnerable target on the legs. It is structurally quite weak and can be attacked from any direction. If you damage your opponent's knee(s), you normally take away that persons ability to maneuver or continue the fight. The kneecap almost always dislocates laterally, so horizontal or 45° angular blows are most efficient. Strikes or pressing attacks to leg nerves will usually weaken the leg or cause a fall. Small fragile foot bones are easily damaged or broken by being stomped on.

Overview

Pressure point fighting is the art of attacking acupoints to assist execution of a technique. In order to understand the use of acupoints in self-defense and combat, it is important to thoroughly review the *Eastern Concepts* chapter, which outlines the basic theories associated with the meridian/acupoint system. The same principles applied to healing, can also be used for destructive purposes. This is the basis of pressure point fighting.

It is important to understand that "combat" is only one aspect of the martial arts, which are also equally concerned with health, wellness, and emotional and spiritual evolution. The principles presented in this section can have significant negative effects on one's health. Be careful, prudent and sensible, and only practice under qualified supervision.

Historical Development

Chinese *Dim Mok*, Korean *Kuepso Chirigi* and Japanese *Atemi* are all systems for attacking the body's vital points. Because these skills were studied in secret until the late twentieth century, the precise origin of these systems is not known, although it is believed that they evolved simultaneously along with healing arts. The earliest surviving documentation comes from China and India. Today, when examining various East Asian systems, we find they are nearly identical, although differences in terminology often disguise this. This similarity is not unexpected, as the human body is essentially the same, regardless of where you live.

Contemporary Approaches

Practical martial arts, such as *Hapkido*, incorporate self-defense techniques that work on several levels: 1) They are effective because they attack anatomically weak areas; 2) Their effectiveness is increased by precisely targeting acupoints in these same regions. For example, kicking the proper acupoint at the knee, will not only disrupt a person's energy, but also break the joint. Most masters begin teaching pressure points at the novice level, gradually revealing more arts over a period of years. Complex or extremely vital points are

rarely taught to students below the black belt level, since most masters do not wish to see knowledge they have spent generations acquiring misused or abused. Also, novices (and many black belts) do not possess the technical proficiency or theoretical understanding of meridian theory to fully and safely exploit its potential—for years they will be struggling with fundamentals, which are far more important and useful anyway. There is also a tradition of secretness in the martial arts, in which *advanced knowledge* was never shared unless a person had proved their loyalty over a long period of time. In many instances, Westerners were completely barred, although this practice is declining.

This practice of guarding proprietary secrets was not only found in the martial arts, but extended into acupuncture and other healing disciplines as well. However, when one observes the history of racism and military conflict which characterized interactions between Asians—and later Westerners and Asians—from the 1500s to the middle of the twentieth century, it is easy to see why these protectionist policies evolved.

Discovering the Secret Arts

The "secret combat arts" which many martial arts claim to possess and jealously guard are, in most cases, not secrets at all. In fact they bare amazing similarity to, and are almost always an extension of, healing theories. If you wish to discover the basis of the pressure point skills used in most martial arts, you must become fluent in the anatomy, physiology and meridian theories associated with the human body. If you can become fluent in an art such as acupuncture, you will be able to discover many of these *secret arts* on your own—simply by applying healing theory in reverse.

The in-depth study of a healing art will also give you a profound respect for health, healing and life that should encourage you to practice the martial arts with a good deal of restraint, compassion and common sense. This is considered an absolute necessity when applying principles outlined in this section.

Attack Purposes

Attacking acupoints can produce several possible results, depending upon the method of attack and individual factors, such as health of opponent, size, susceptibility, etc.:

- Pain
- Immediate involuntary reactions
- Delayed reactions (minutes, hours, days)
- Paralysis
- Disorientation (dazed, stunned)
- Loss of consciousness (momentary)
- Loss of consciousness (extended)
- Death
- Nothing (attack is ineffective)

ATTACK PRINCIPLES

Several basic principles are applied when executing acupoint attacks. These principles are derived from acupuncture and basically employ healing theory for destructive purposes. When examining acupoint attacks in most martial arts, you will find that they usually correspond with one or more of these principles. Basic attack principles are listed below and outlined on the following pages.

1. Attack points sensitive to pressure
2. Attack multiple points in the same area
3. Attack both bilateral points
4. Attack a meridian at multiple points
5. Attack related meridians (yin/yang pairs)
6. Attack according to Qi-flow timing
7. Attack using conquest cycle (5 phases)
8. Attack Special Acupoints

Importance of Accuracy

The previous principles depend on accuracy. Attacking an acupoint requires very precise targeting, usually combined with a specific angle of attack. If targeting is off by a half inch, the point may be unaffected. If targeting is correct, but the angle incorrect, the point will again be unaffected. Movement, clothing and other factors all influence your ability to accurately target points. Remember, finding acupoints on yourself or a helpful partner is very different than hitting a moving target, particularly if acupoints lie hidden beneath clothing, or are protected by padding.

1. Attack Points Sensitive to Pressure

The clearest, fastest and most consistent responses are achieved by attacking sensitive acupoints located on major nerves. Pain produces immediate involuntary reactions in almost all people, particularly when the attack is unexpected. Results can range from involuntary muscle responses and partial loss of motor functions (from damage to nerves serving muscles), to loss of consciousness (for reasons which remain unclear, but hint at neural involvement). Acupoint strikes that affect nerves are usually used to make an opponent release a hold; lead an opponent into a technique you wish to apply, such as a hold or throw; or impair an attacker's ability to continue fighting. Heavily muscled individuals are often more sensitive to acupoint pressure than flabby persons. This is because developed muscles tend to tighten the space around the points, pushing them in against the bone or outward towards the surface.

Typical Examples

Many acupoints are sensitive to pressure. A few of the more common ones are:

- GB-41 on foot
- TW-23 on temple
- CO-17 on chest
- SP-10 above knee
- TW-11 at back of elbow
- LI-4 between thumb and index finger
- GB-31 on upper-outer leg
- GV-26 between nose and lip (see below)

2. Attack Multiple Points in Same Area

Stimulation of an acupoint manipulates Qi-flow in the *immediate area,* thereby affecting surrounding muscles, tissue, joints or organs. Striking multiple points in the same region will compound this effect. This can involve a single blow to two or more closely placed points, multiple blows to different points, or repeated blows to the same point. Be aware that closely placed points must sometimes be attacked from different directions, thus requiring multiple strikes, since a single strike would affect only one point.

Typical Examples

- Strike TW-10 and TW-11 behind the elbow, using two blows, to weaken the arm and hand. These acupoints are about 1 inch apart.

- Strike LU-5, M-UE-31 and M-UE-32 on the inner forearm (thumb side), using a single blow. The most common method is to use a Raking Back Fist or Forearm Strike directed toward the hand. To increase its effectiveness, practitioners often hold and press a Lung or Pericardium acupoint on the wrist, thereby increasing the number of points attacked. This strike is typically found in basic Hapkido defenses against a clothing grab.

- Strike SP-12 and LV-12 in the inguinal (groin) region, using one or more blows. This is often used to bring the head forward, or execute a throw against a kick (see below).

3. Attack Both Bilateral Points

Bilateral acupoints occur symmetrically on the left and right sides of the body. The majority of acupoints are bilateral, including all those located on the 12 Regular meridians. When attacking a single bilateral point, the opposing meridian is believed to partially compensate for the disruption. An attack to both bilateral points is believed to be particularly disruptive to Qi and neurological functions, since both meridians on opposing sides are affected. When special points are used, bilateral strikes can cause disorientation and loss of consciousness, often with minimal force. Strikes to multiple pairs of bilateral points increase the effect of a blow.

Be very careful when applying the examples below and practice only under supervised instruction. During practice, strikes to both bilateral points are usually only articulated, with no contact being made.

Typical Examples

- Strike diagonally upward to both LV-13 points at the ribs, using the points of your knuckles.

- Strike HT-1 points in both armpits using the fingertips of both hands (usually against a front choke).

- Strike LI-18 points at both sides of the neck, using the tips of both thumbs. Hit straight inward from both sides toward opposing points (see below).

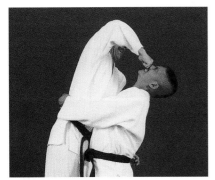

*1. Attack points sensitive to pressure
(fore-knuckle press to GV-26 between nose and lip)*

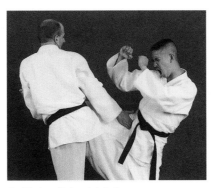

*2. Attack multiple points in the same area
(Spear Hand to SP-12 and LV-12 in inguinal region)*

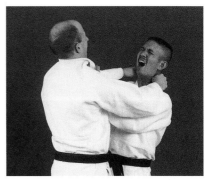

*3. Attack both bilateral points
(Twin Thumb Hands to LI-18 at sides of neck)*

4. Attack a Meridian at Multiple Points

The effectiveness of an attack is increased by striking one or more points on the same meridian, usually on the same side of the body. Most attacks begin at the outer extremities (hand, leg) and work inward toward the chest or head, finishing at the first or last meridian point, which is considered more sensitive. Once the first point is struck, the meridian becomes activated, and the second point can often be struck minutes later with the same effect (depending on Qi-flow timing).

Typical Examples

• An attacker grabs your wrist or belt with their palm facing down. Using your knuckles, strike a TW acupoint on the back of the hand (TW-2 or TW-3), or above the wrist (TW-4, 5, 6, 7, or 8), depending on what is most exposed. You may even use a raking strike (e.g., Back Fist) to hit several points on the first blow. Follow with a strike to TW-17 behind the ear, or TW-23 at the temple.

• An attacker delivers a straight knife thrust to your face. Execute a block (using your wrist) to a cluster of four acupoints located on the wrist along the ulnar nerve (HT-4, 5, 6, 7); followed by an almost simultaneous Front Toe Kick into the armpit (HT-1), where the brachial plexus branches into major nerves serving the arm and chest (see below). This strike *should not* be practiced on individuals with known or suspected heart conditions.

5. Attack Related Meridians

The 12 Regular meridians are sequentially linked and grouped in six yin/yang pairs (LU-LI; ST-SP; HT-SI; BL-KI; PC-TW; GB-LV). This pairing corresponds to the flow of Qi. Attacking points on two or more related meridians is believed to be disruptive to the flow of Qi, distorting the balance of yin and yang forces within the body (physically weakening the opponent). Although this rationale is "very traditional", specific cause-and-effect relationships have been consistently noted by Eastern medical practitioners and martial artists across a variety of systems and styles.

Typical Examples

• Grab and press HT-2 or HT-3 near the elbow, while your other hand executes a hooking thumb-knuckle strike to SI-16 at the side of the neck. Strike at a 45° angle to the neck, from back to front.

• Stomp GB-41 (top of foot) using your toe, heel, or the edge of your shoe, then hit LV-14 at the ribs with the point of your knuckle. This strike could also be used against an opponent holding you with a bear-hug from behind.

• Strike SP-21 at the side of the trunk using a hooking punch (hit with the point of knuckle); followed by a Palm Heel Strike to ST-5 at the notch on the bottom of the jaw, hitting 45° upward from the side. This combination can also be executed simultaneously (see below).

6. Attack According Qi-Flow Timing

Qi flows through the 12 Regular meridians in prescribed order and timing, based on a 24-hour cycle. Each meridian is "active" for two hours every day, which is the period when Qi is most concentrated. Attacking a meridian during its active period will magnify the effect of acupoint strikes. Attacking a meridian during its most dormant period (12 hours later), is much less effective, but may produce effects that manifest themselves when the meridian is again active, 12 hours later. When the Qi is moving between two sequential meridians (e.g., Gallbladder and Liver), attacks to acupoints on both meridians would be very effective, particularly if they are yin-yang pairs. The chart in the *Eastern Concepts* chapter, under *Meridians,* outlines Qi-flow timing and sequence.

Typical Examples

• From 9 pm to 11 pm, strikes to points on the Triple Warmer meridian are more effective.

• Around 11 pm, Qi is moving between the Triple Warmer and Gallbladder meridians (yang-yang), suggesting attacks to acupoints on either one or both meridians.

• Around 1 am, Qi is moving between the Gallbladder and Liver meridians (a yang-yin pair), suggesting attacks to acupoints on both meridians (see below). This last example also makes use of the previous principle, "*attack related meridians.*"

4. Attack a Meridian at Multiple Points
(Bent-Wrist Block to HT-4, Front Toe Kick to HT-1)

5. Attack Related Meridians
(Middle Finger Fist to SP-21, Palm Heel to ST-5)

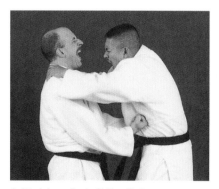

6. Attack According to Qi-Flow Timing
(1 am: Twin Uppercut to GB-24 and LV-14, at rib cage)

7. Attack Using the Conquest Cycle

As explained in the Philosophy chapter, the *five phase theory* (wood, fire, earth, metal, water) was used by ancient East Asians to develop a system of cyclical patterns and correspondences, within which all natural phenomena were organized. Thus, each of the 12 Regular meridians are associated with a particular phase (e.g., Lung is metal). The five phases can be sequentially ordered into 36 possible cyclical patterns. The most important pattern for combat is called the *conquest cycle,* in which phases follow a *destructive* sequence: wood > earth > water > fire > metal. In the conquest cycle: wood conquers earth, earth conquers water, water conquers fire, fire conquers metal, metal conquers wood, repeating the cycle again.

In ancient martial arts, the conquest cycle was originally used to map correspondences between meridian acupoints, to prioritize strike selection. For example, a strike to the Liver meridian (wood) might be followed by an attack to the Stomach meridian (earth), thus completing one step in the conquest cycle (wood conquers earth). If the previous combination were followed by an attack to the Kidney meridian (water), a second step in the conquest cycle would be completed (earth conquers water). The effectiveness of combinations increases as more steps in the conquest cycle are completed. Historically, a completed cycle comprised of five such acupoint attacks was considered lethal.

Today, five phase theory and the conquest cycle is best used as a simplistic way to remember meridian relationships, and as a theoretical context for understanding the evolution of acupoint combinations used in combat. If one bases acupoint choice totally on a mechanical application of the conquest cycle, they are likely to be disappointed by the results. In contemporary Eastern medicine, this type of antiquated approach is actively discouraged. The chart below shows common meridian striking sequences based on the conquest cycle. Use this as a starting point for creating pressure point combinations.

Typical Example
- Strike LV-13 (wood) at ribs with your knuckles (at an upward angle). Strike ST-9 (earth) at side of neck with your knuckles or a thrusting Knife Hand (at a 45° angle front to back). In this sequence, wood conquers earth.

Meridian Sequences Based on Conquest Cycle

Phase	Sequences	Sequences
Wood	Liver	Gallbladder
Earth	Stomach	Stomach
Water	Bladder	Kidney
Fire	Heart	Pericardium
Metal	Lung	Large Intestine
Wood	Liver	Gallbladder
Earth	Stomach	Stomach
Water	Kidney	Kidney
Fire	Heart	Pericardium
Metal	Large Intestine	Large Intestine
Wood	Liver	Gallbladder
Earth	Spleen	Spleen
Water	Bladder	Bladder
Fire	Pericardium	Triple Warmer
Metal	Lung	Large Intestine
Wood	Liver	Gallbladder
Earth	Spleen	Spleen
Water	Kidney	Kidney
Fire	Triple Warmer	Small Intestine
Metal	Lung	Large Intestine

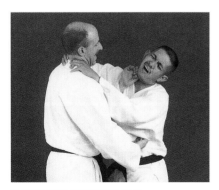

7. Attack Using the Conquest Cycle
(Knuckle Fist to LV-13 at ribs, Knuckle Hand to ST-9)

8. Attack Special Acupoints

The effectiveness of an acupoint attack is increased by striking acupoints that belong to "Special Acupoint Groupings." These groupings and their unique characteristics were covered previously. The most commonly used groupings include Source Points, Alarm Points, Connecting Points, Associated Points and Intersection Points. Strikes to one or more special points may also involve many of the other attack principles previously covered.

Typical Example
- Strike four special points below the navel, with a single punch (directed diagonally up or down). These points span about 2.5 inches. Both CO-3 and CO-4 are Intersection Points for the SP, KI, PC, and LV meridians; and Alarm Points for the BL and SI meridians. CO-5 is an Alarm Point for TW meridian. CO-6 is the body's Qi center.

- Strike LV-3 on the top of the foot using your knuckle or the corner of your shoe heel (diagonally downward). This acupoint is the Source Point for the Liver meridian.

- Strike CO-17 at the sternum using your knuckle (straight punch, see below). CO-17 is an extremely vital target; it is an Intersection Point of four meridians (SP, SI, KI, TW), an Alarm Point for the Pericardium, and one of the eight important points influencing Qi (Meeting-Hui Point). It also lies near the heart and should not be struck during practice.

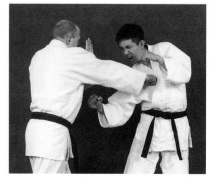

8. Attack Special Acupoints
(Middle Finger Fist to CO-17 at sternum)

MAJOR PRESSURE POINT TARGETS

The illustrations below and on subsequent pages, show the basic acupoint targets commonly used in many martial arts; many others are also used (see *Acupoint Charts*). However location, function and use of these basic acupoints should be learned before proceeding further. Remember, it is better to become highly proficient in a few techniques, than marginally competent with many.

The next two pages describe the effects historically associated with specific acupoint attacks. It is important to realize that clinical testing to verify these results has never occurred, for obvious reasons: willing victims are not lining up for testing. Historically, loss of consciousness, impaired motor functions, death and other strike effects were primarily attributed to disruption of Qi-flow, although the following anatomical and physiological damage has also been noted:

Head Area

Strikes to most acupoints located on the head will cause trauma to cranial nerves or the brain, resulting in varying degrees of loss of coordination, disruption of sensory and motor functions, vascular shock, and loss of consciousness. They do not normally lead to stoppage of breathing. Strikes to the following acupoints have been most consistently associated with loss of consciousness:

BL-10	SI-18	TW-23
GB-13 to 15	ST-5	
GB-20	ST-7	

Neck Area

Strikes to acupoints on the neck can cause trauma to the carotid artery and a variety of cranial and cervical nerves, resulting in shock, loss of sensory and motor functions, and eventually leading to loss of consciousness. The following acupoints have been most consistently associated with loss of consciousness:

CO-22	SI-17	TW-17
LI-18	ST-9	
SI-16	ST-10	

CO-22 (Sternal Notch)

Straight strikes can damage the trachea and obstruct the airway, resulting in death unless breathing functions are immediately restored by emergency surgery. Pressing attacks directed inward and down may cause loss of consciousness without damaging the trachea. This is usually accomplished by thrusting with the tips of your index and middle fingers.

Chest and Abdomen

Strikes to acupoints located on the trunk will cause trauma to internal organs and produce disruptive effects on the nervous system. This subsequently affects cranial nerves, resulting in shock and loss of sensory and motor functions, eventually leading to loss of consciousness and breathing functions. This then leads to circulatory failure and death unless breathing is restored. Possible effects linked to specific points include:

CO-17 (Sternum), KI-23 (Over Heart)

Strikes to these acupoints can result in cardiac irregularities or failure, particularly in individuals with weak hearts.

LU-1, ST-17, PC-1 (Chest)

Strikes to these points disrupt the respiratory system. Blows to acupoints above and below the nipple (ST-16 and ST-18) also work well.

CO-15 (Xiphoid Process)

Strikes to this point may cause severe trauma to the liver, stomach and heart and produce disruptive effects on the nervous system.

CO-2, 3, 4, 5, 6 (Below Navel)

Strikes directed to these points can cause trauma to the small intestine and bladder, affecting the blood vessels and nerves in the abdomen, which results in shock and loss of motor functions.

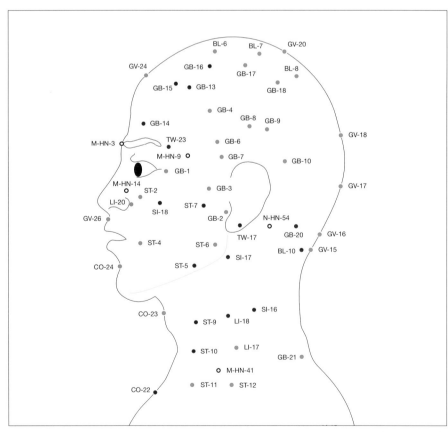

Pressure point targets on the head and neck (red indicates points most consistently linked to loss of consciousness).

Groin (Inguinal Crease)

Strikes to SP-12 and LV-12 will cause trauma to a variety of nerves and blood vessels (see *Meridian Reference*) often producing pain in the hip and abdomen. Powerful blows can cause loss of motor functions and sometimes loss of consciousness.

Side of Thigh

Strikes to GB-31 and GB-32 in the vastus lateralis muscle causes trauma to the lateral femoral cutaneous nerve and muscular branch of the femoral nerve, leading to cramping of the thigh muscles and subsequent loss of motor functions in the leg. Pain in the abdomen is sometimes present.

Knee

Strikes to acupoints at the knee (e.g., SP-9, SP-10, ST-34, N-LE-7) are used to impair mobility, cause pain, or dislocate the kneecap.

Lower Leg

Strikes to SP-6 and LV-6 on the inner shin, and GB-41 and LV-3 on the foot, cause trauma to nerves and arteries, weakening the leg and sometimes causing pain in the leg, hip or abdomen area.

Closely Spaced Acupoints

The following acupoints are often attacked simultaneously using a single strike, since they are very close together. Always use a hitting surface that corresponds to point placement and local anatomy.

Point Group	Region	Typical Attack Point
BL-13, 14, 15	Back	Knuckle Fist, Ox Jaw Hand
CO-3, 4, 5, 6	Belly	Fore Fist (down or upward)
CO-22, ST-11	Neck	Pincer Hand, Spear Hand
GB-8, GB-9	Head	Knuckle Fist
GB-13, GB-15	Head	Palm Heel, Back Fist
GB-24, LV-14	Ribs	Knuckle Hand
HT-4, 5, 6, 7	Arm	Back Fist, Bent Wrist
LU-5, M-UE-31 and M-UE-32	Arm	Raking Back Fist
LV-12, SP-12	Groin	Spear Hand
PC-1, ST-17	Chest	Knuckle Fist, Fore Fist
ST-9, ST-10	Neck	Knuckle Hand, Ridge Hand
ST-11, M-HN-41	Neck	Pincer Hand

Safe Practice Sessions

Since pressure point strikes basically employ healing principles for destructive purposes, even light training poses a certain element of risk. The effects of constant, long-term practice are not known. Since neurological involvement is suspected, but has not been medically verified, be aware of possible long-term negative effects on health. Progressive neurological damage, negative biochemical changes, and Qi blockages may contribute to a variety of unhealthy conditions in the body, which may lead to serious medical problems. These and many other questions remain unanswered. For this reason, the following precautions are suggested when training with partners:

- Learn basic healing and revival principles first; only practice under qualified supervision.

- Limit practice time to once a week or less.

- Do not strike both bilateral points; limit practice sessions to one side of body.

- Strike or press lightly. It is not necessary to hammer someone to gauge the effect of a technique.

- If someone experiences dizziness, disorientation, persistent pain, etc., discontinue practice and seek qualified medical attention.

- Do not practice on individuals with medical or psychological problems, persons on medication, or in poor physical condition. Exercise greater caution with older persons.

- After practicing acupoint attacks, use meditation, acupressure or other body balancing techniques to restore the body's normal healthy state. Do this regardless of how you feel. It certainly can't hurt.

Loss of Consciousness

It is not uncommon for breathing or heart functions to cease when a person is rendered unconscious. This may result from a choke hold cutting off the air or blood supply (common in Judo competitions), or by striking certain acupoints, singly or in combination. This can occur with a minimal amount of force, sometimes unintentionally, particularly when acupoints are accurately targeted. Restoration of breathing and heart functions is often quite simple for someone with proper medical training. For someone without training, or in the absence of immediate attention, an individual might easily die or suffer permanent brain damage.

Therefore, unless someone present is trained in CPR or other appropriate revival procedures, you would be wise to refrain from "risky" practice. Use of accepted Eastern revival techniques in the United States, which are well established and proven in Asia, may leave you vulnerable to a lawsuit, since they are not currently approved by the American Medical Association. Such revival techniques are outlined in an earlier chapter. CPR and other Western emergency medical procedures are easily learned and frequently taught for free at the community level.

Final Thoughts

Many within the martial arts community believe that future innovations in the martial arts will be intimately linked to an increased understanding of the human body. This ever-expanding body of knowledge should improve training methods and body care, while also facilitating development of more efficient, safer and gentler techniques for controlling individuals.

The application of acupoints and meridian theory to self-defense situations, has tremendous implications for women and smaller individuals, who would normally be overwhelmed by much larger opponents, regardless of their skill level. An attacker's size, weight, speed and power can quickly negate your technique, even if it is vastly superior. Many black belts are genuinely shocked the first time this happens to them in a real confrontation. The application of meridian theory to self-defense situations affords an opportunity to make these confrontations more equal.

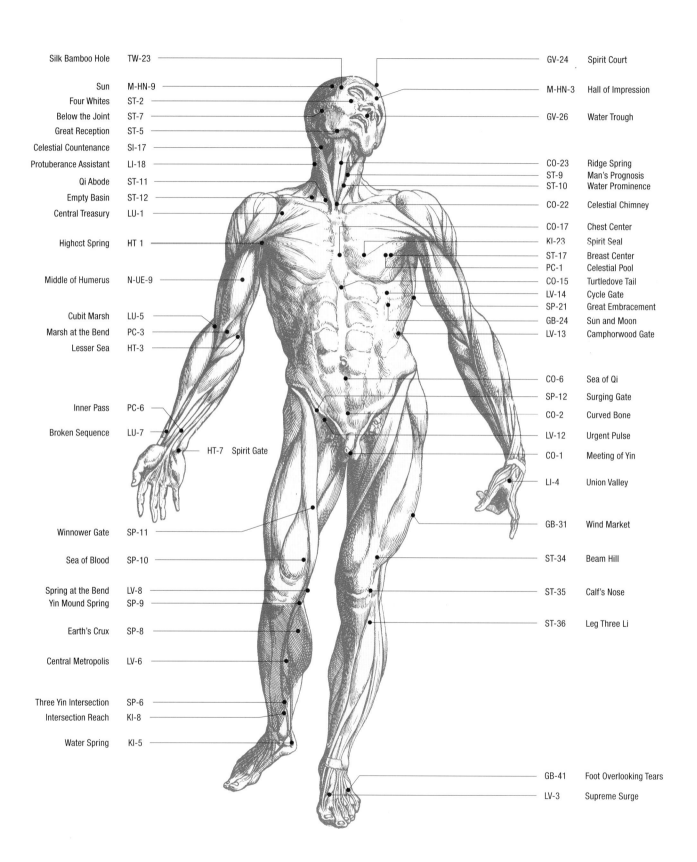

Silk Bamboo Hole	TW-23
Sun	M-HN-9
Four Whites	ST-2
Below the Joint	ST-7
Great Reception	ST-5
Celestial Countenance	SI-17
Protuberance Assistant	LI-18
Qi Abode	ST-11
Empty Basin	ST-12
Central Treasury	LU-1
Highest Spring	HT 1
Middle of Humerus	N-UE-9
Cubit Marsh	LU-5
Marsh at the Bend	PC-3
Lesser Sea	HT-3
Inner Pass	PC-6
Broken Sequence	LU-7
HT-7	Spirit Gate
Winnower Gate	SP-11
Sea of Blood	SP-10
Spring at the Bend	LV-8
Yin Mound Spring	SP-9
Earth's Crux	SP-8
Central Metropolis	LV-6
Three Yin Intersection	SP-6
Intersection Reach	KI-8
Water Spring	KI-5

GV-24	Spirit Court
M-HN-3	Hall of Impression
GV-26	Water Trough
CO-23	Ridge Spring
ST-9	Man's Prognosis
ST-10	Water Prominence
CO-22	Celestial Chimney
CO-17	Chest Center
KI-23	Spirit Seal
ST-17	Breast Center
PC-1	Celestial Pool
CO-15	Turtledove Tail
LV-14	Cycle Gate
SP-21	Great Embracement
GB-24	Sun and Moon
LV-13	Camphorwood Gate
CO-6	Sea of Qi
SP-12	Surging Gate
CO-2	Curved Bone
LV-12	Urgent Pulse
CO-1	Meeting of Yin
LI-4	Union Valley
GB-31	Wind Market
ST-34	Beam Hill
ST-35	Calf's Nose
ST-36	Leg Three Li
GB-41	Foot Overlooking Tears
LV-3	Supreme Surge

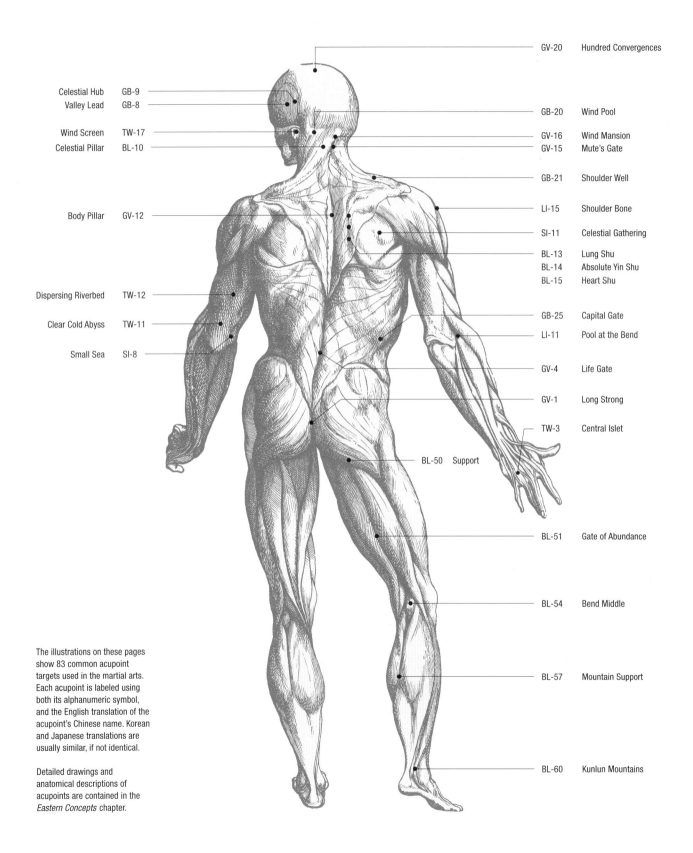

GV-20   Hundred Convergences

Celestial Hub   GB-9

Valley Lead   GB-8

GB-20   Wind Pool

Wind Screen   TW-17

GV-16   Wind Mansion

Celestial Pillar   BL-10

GV-15   Mute's Gate

GB-21   Shoulder Well

LI-15   Shoulder Bone

Body Pillar   GV-12

SI-11   Celestial Gathering

BL-13   Lung Shu

BL-14   Absolute Yin Shu

BL-15   Heart Shu

Dispersing Riverbed   TW-12

GB-25   Capital Gate

Clear Cold Abyss   TW-11

LI-11   Pool at the Bend

Small Sea   SI-8

GV-4   Life Gate

GV-1   Long Strong

TW-3   Central Islet

BL-50   Support

BL-51   Gate of Abundance

BL-54   Bend Middle

The illustrations on these pages show 83 common acupoint targets used in the martial arts. Each acupoint is labeled using both its alphanumeric symbol, and the English translation of the acupoint's Chinese name. Korean and Japanese translations are usually similar, if not identical.

BL-57   Mountain Support

Detailed drawings and anatomical descriptions of acupoints are contained in the *Eastern Concepts* chapter.

BL-60   Kunlun Mountains

A

An Mian 安眠 N-HN-54

B

Ba Xie 八邪 M-UE-22
Bai Huan Shu 白環俞 BL-30
Bai Hui 百會 GV-20
Bai Lao 百勞 M-HN-30
Ban Men 板門 M-UE-13
Bao Huang 胞肓 BL-48 [53]
Ben Shen 本神 GB-13
Bi Guan 臂關 ST-31
Bi Nao 臂臑 LI-14
Bi Tong 鼻通 M-HN-14
Bi Zhong 臂中 M-UE-30
Bing Feng 秉風 SI-12
Bu Lang 步廊 KI-22
Bu Rong 不容 ST-19

C

Chang Qiang 長強 GV-1
Cheng Fu 承扶 BL-50 [36]
Cheng Guang 承光 BL-6
Cheng Jiang 承漿 CO-24
Cheng Jin 承筋 BL-56
Cheng Ling 承靈 GB-18
Cheng Man 承滿 ST-20
Cheng Qi 承泣 ST-1
Cheng Shan 承山 BL-57
Chi Mai 瘈脈 TW-18
Chi Ze 尺澤 LU-5
Chong Gu 崇骨 M-HN-31
Chong Men 沖門 SP-12
Chong Yang 沖陽 ST-42
Ci Liao 次髎 BL-32

D

Da Bao 大胞 SP-21
Da Chang Shu 大腸俞 BL-25
Da Du 大都 SP-2
Da Dun 大敦 LV-1
Da He 大赫 KI-12
Da Heng 大橫 SP-15
Da Ju 大巨 ST-27
Da Ling 大陵 PC-7
Da Ying 大迎 ST-5
Da Zhong 大鐘 KI-4
Da Zhu 大杼 BL-11
Da Zhui 大椎 GV-14
Dai Mai 帶脈 GB-26
Dan Nang Xue 膽囊穴 M-LE-23
Dan Shu 膽俞 BL-19
Di Cang 地倉 ST-4
Di Ji 地機 SP-8
Di Wu Hui 地五會 GB-42
Ding Shu 疔俞 M-UE-28
Du Bi 犢鼻 ST-35
Du Shu 督俞 BL-16
Dui Duan 兌端 GV-27

E

Er Bai 二白 M-UE-29
Er Jian 二間 LI-2
Er Men 耳門 TW-21

F

Fei Shu 肺俞 BL-13
Fei Yang 飛揚 BL-58
Feng Chi 風池 GB-20
Feng Fu 風府 GV-16
Feng Long 豐隆 ST-40
Feng Men 風門 BL-12
Feng Shi 風市 GB-31
Fu Ai 腹哀 SP-16

Fu Bai 浮白 GB-10
Fu Fen 附分 BL-36 [41]
Fu Jie 腹結 SP-14
Fu Liu 復溜 KI-7
Fu She 府舍 SP-13
Fu Tú 扶突 LI-18
Fu Tù 伏兔 ST-32
Fu Xi 浮郄 BL-52 [38]
Fu Yang 跗陽 BL-59

G

Gan Shu 肝俞 BL-18
Gao Huang Shu 膏肓俞 BL-38 [43]
Ge Guan 膈關 BL-41 [46]
Ge Shu 膈俞 BL-17
Gen Jin 跟緊 N-LE-9
Gen Ping 跟平 N-LE-3
Gong Sun 公孫 SP-4
Gong Zhong 肱中 N-UE-9
Guan Chong 關衝 TW-1
Guan Men 關門 ST-22
Guan Yuan 關元 CO-4
Guan Yuan Shu 關元俞 BL-26
Guang Ming 光明 GB-37
Gui Lai 歸來 ST-29

H

Han Yan 頷厭 GB-4
He Gu 合谷 LI-4
He Liao 禾髎 LI-19
He Liao 和髎 TW-22
He Yang 合陽 BL-55
Heng Gu 橫骨 KI-11
Hou Ding 後頂 GV-19
Hou Xi 後谿 SI-3
Hu Bian 虎邊 N-UE-15
Hua Gai 華蓋 CO-20
Hua Rou Men 滑肉門 ST-24

Huan Tiao 環跳 GB-30
Huang Men 肓門 BL-46 51
Huang Shu 肓俞 KI-16
Hui Yang 會陽 BL-35
Hui Yin 會陰 CO-1
Hui Zong 會宗 TW-7
Hun Men 魂門 BL-42 47

J

Ji Mai 急脈 LV-12
Ji Men 箕門 SP-11
Ji Quan 極泉 HT-1
Ji Zhong 脊中 GV-6
Jia Che 頰車 ST-6
Jia Ji 夾脊 M-BW-35
Jia Xi 夾谿 GB-43
Jian Jing 肩井 GB-21
Jian Li 建里 CO-11
Jian Liao 肩髎 TW-14
Jian Nei Ling 肩內陵 M-UE-48
Jian Shi 間使 PC-5
Jian Wai Shu 肩外俞 SI-14
Jian Yu 肩髃 LI-15
Jian Zhen 肩貞 SI-9
Jian Zhong Shu 肩中俞 SI-15
Jiao Sun 角孫 TW-20
Jiao Xin 交信 KI-8
Jie Xi 解谿 ST-41
Jin Men 金門 BL-63
Jin Suo 筋縮 GV-8
Jing Bi 頸臂 M-HN-41
Jing Gu 京骨 BL-64
Jing Men 京門 GB-25
Jing Ming 睛明 BL-1
Jing Qu 經渠 LU-8
Jiu Wei 鳩尾 CO-15
Ju Gu 巨骨 LI-16
Ju Liao (face) 巨髎 ST-3

Ju Liao (hip) 居髎 GB-29
Ju Que 巨闕 CO-14
Jue Gu* 絕骨 GB-39
Jue Yin Shu 厥陰俞 BL-14

K

Kong Zui 孔最 LU-6
Ku Fang 庫房 ST-14
Kun Lun 昆侖 BL-60

L

Lan Wei Xue 闌尾穴 M-LE-13
Lao Gong 勞宮 PC-8
Li Dui 厲兌 ST-45
Li Gou 蠡溝 LV-5
Li Wai 里外 N-LE-7
Lian Quan 廉泉 CO-23
Liang Men 梁門 ST-21
Liang Qiu 梁丘 ST-34
Lie Que 列缺 LU-7
Lin Qi (foot) 臨泣 (足) GB-41
Ling Dao 靈道 HT-4
Ling Tai 靈台 GV-10
Ling Xu 靈墟 KI-24
Lou Gu 漏谷 SP-7
Lu Xi 顱息 TW-19
Luo Que 絡卻 BL-8
Luo Zhen 落枕 M-UE-24

M

Mei Chong 眉衝 BL-3
Ming Men 命門 GV-4
Mu Chuang 目窗 GB-16

N

Nao Hu 腦戶 GV-17
Nao Hui 腦會 TW-13
Nao Kong 腦空 GB-19

Nao Shang 臑上 N-UE-14
Nao Shu 臑俞 SI-10
Nei Guan 內關 PC-6
Nei Ting 內庭 ST-44

P

Pang Guang Shu 膀胱俞 BL-28
Pi Gen 痞根 M-BW-16
Pi Shu 脾俞 BL-20
Pian Li 偏歷 LI-6
Po Hu 魄戶 BL-37 42
Pu Can 僕參 BL-61

Q

Qi Chong 氣沖 ST-30
Qi Hai 氣海 CO-6
Qi Hai Shu 氣海俞 BL-24
Qi Hu 氣戶 ST-13
Qi Men 期門 LV-14
Qi She 氣舍 ST-11
Qi Xue 氣穴 KI-13
Qian Ding 前頂 GV-21
Qian Gu 前谷 SI-2
Qiang Jian 強間 GV-18
Qiao Yin (foot) 竅陰 (足) GB-44
Qing Leng Yuan 清冷淵 TW-11
Qing Ling 青靈 HT-2
Qiu Xu 丘墟 GB-40
Qu Bin 曲鬢 GB-7
Qu Chai 曲差 BL-4
Qu Chi 曲池 LI-11
Qu Gu 曲骨 CO-2
Qu Quan 曲泉 LV-8
Qu Yuan 曲垣 SI-13
Qu Ze 曲澤 PC-3
Quan Liao 顴髎 SI-18
Que Pen 缺盆 ST-12

R

Ran Gu　然谷　KI-2
Ren Ying　人迎　ST-9
Ren Zhong*　人中　GV-26
Ri Yue　日月　GB-24
Ru Gen　乳根　ST-18
Ru Zhong　乳中　ST-17

S

San Jian　三間　LI-3
San Jiao Shu　三焦俞　BL-22
San Yang Luo　三陽絡　TW-8
San Yin Jiao　三陰交　SP-6
Shan Ge　山根　M-HN-4
Shan Zhong　膻中　CO-17
Shang Ba Xie　上八邪　M-UE-50
Shang Guǎn*　上管　CO-13
Shang Guān　上關　GB-3
Shang Ju Xu　上巨虛　ST-37
Shang Lian　上廉　LI-9
Shang Liao　上膠　BL-31
Shang Qiu　商丘　SP-5
Shang Qu　商曲　KI-17
Shang Wan　上脘　CO-13
Shang Xing　上星　GV-23
Shang Yang　商陽　LI-1
Shao Chong　少沖　HT-9
Shao Fu　少府　HT-8
Shao Hai　少海　HT-3
Shao Shang　少商　LU-11
Shao Ze　少澤　SI-1
Shen Cang　神藏　KI-25
Shen Dao　神道　GV-11
Shen Feng　神封　KI-23
Shen Mai　申脈　BL-62
Shen Men　神門　HT-7
Shen Que　神闕　CO-8
Shen Shu　腎俞　BL-23

Shen Tang　神堂　BL-39 [44]
Shen Ting　神庭　GV-24
Shen Zhu　身柱　GV-12
Shi Dou　食竇　SP-17
Shi Guan　石關　KI-18
Shi Men　石門　CO-5
Shi Qi Zhui Xia　十七椎下　M-BW-25
Shou San Li　手三里　LI-10
Shou Wu Li　手五里　LI-13
Shu Fu　俞府　KI-27
Shu Gu　束骨　BL-65
Shuai Gu　率谷　GB-8
Shui Dao　水道　ST-28
Shui Fen　水分　CO-9
Shui Gou　水溝　GV-26
Shui Quan　水泉　KI-5
Shui Tu　水突　ST-10
Si Bai　四白　ST-2
Si Du　四瀆　TW-9
Si Man　四滿　KI-14
Si Shen Cong　四神聰　M-HN-1
Si Zhu Kong　絲竹空　TW-23
Su Liao　素膠　GV-25

T

Tai Bai　太白　SP-3
Tai Chong　太沖　LV-3
Tai Xi　太谿　KI-3
Tai Yang　太陽　M-HN-9
Tai Yi　太乙　ST-23
Tai Yuan　太淵　LU-9
Tao Dao　陶道　GV-13
Tian Chi　天池　PC-1
Tian Chong　天衝　GB-9
Tian Chuang　天窗　SI-16
Tian Ding　天鼎　LI-17
Tian Fu　天府　LU-3
Tian Jing　天井　TW-10

Tian Liao　天膠　TW-15
Tian Quan　天泉　PC-2
Tian Rong　天容　SI-17
Tian Shu　天樞　ST-25
Tian Tu　天突　CO-22
Tian Xi　天谿　SP-18
Tian You　天牖　TW-16
Tian Zhu　天柱　BL-10
Tian Zong　天宗　SI-11
Tiao Kou　條口　ST-38
Ting Gong　聽宮　SI-19
Ting Hui　聽會　GB-2
Tong Gu　通谷　BL-66
Tong Gu　通谷　KI-20
Tong Li　通里　HT-5
Tong Tian　通天　BL-7
Tong Zi Liao　瞳子膠　GB-1
Tou Lin Qi　頭臨泣　GB-15
Tou Qiao Yin　頭竅陰　GB-11
Tou Wei　頭維　ST-8

W

Wai Guan　外關　TW-5
Wai Ling　外陵　ST-26
Wai Qiu　外丘　GB-36
Wán Gu　完骨　GB-12
Wàn Gu　腕骨　SI-4
Wei Cang　胃倉　BL-45 [50]
Wei Dao　維道　GB-28
Wei Shu　胃俞　BL-21
Wei Yang　委陽　BL-53 [39]
Wei Zhong　委中　BL-54 [40]
Wen Liu　溫溜　LI-7
Wu Chu　五處　BL-5
Wu Li (arm)　五里 (手)　LI-13
Wu Li (foot)　五里 (足)　LV-10
Wu Shu　五樞　GB-27
Wu Yi　屋翳　ST-15

X

Xi Guan　膝關　LV-7
Xi Men　郄門　PC-4
Xi Yan　膝眼　M-LE-16
Xi Yang Guan　膝陽關　GB-33
Xia Bai　俠白　LU-4
Xia Guǎn*　下管　CO-10
Xia Guān　下關　ST-7
Xia Ju Xu　下巨虛　ST-39
Xia Lian　下廉　LI-8
Xia Liao　下髎　BL-34
Xia Wan　下脘　CO-10
Xian Gu　陷谷　ST-43
Xiao Chang Shu　小腸俞　BL-27
Xiao Hai　小海　SI-8
Xiao Luo　消濼　TW-12
Xin Hui　囟會　GV-22
Xin Shi　新識　M-HN-29
Xin Shu　心俞　BL-15
Xing Jian　行間　LV-2
Xiong Xiang　胸鄉　SP-19
Xuan Ji　璇璣　CO-21
Xuan Li　懸厘　GB-6
Xuan Lu　懸顱　GB-5
Xuan Shu　懸樞　GV-5
Xuan Zhong　懸鐘　GB-39
Xue Hai　血海　SP-10

Y

Ya Men　啞門　GV-15
Yang Bai　陽白　GB-14
Yang Chi　陽池　TW-4
Yang Fu　陽輔　GB-38
Yang Gang　陽綱　BL-43 [48]
Yang Gu　陽谷　SI-5
Yang Guān　陽關　GV-3
Yang Guān (knee)　陽關 (膝)　GB-33
Yang Jiao　陽交　GB-35

Yang Lao　養老　SI-6
Yang Ling Quan　陽陵泉　GB-34
Yang Xi　陽谿　LI-5
Yao Shu　腰俞　GV-2
Yao Tong #1　腰痛1　N-UE-19a
Yao Tong #2　腰痛2　N-UE-19b
Yao Tong #3　腰痛3　N-UE-19c
Yao Yan　腰眼　M-BW-24
Yao Yang Guan　腰陽關　GV-3
Ye Men　液門　TW-2
Yi Feng　翳風　TW-17
Yi She　意舍　BL-44 [49]
Yi Xi　譩譆　BL-40 [45]
Yin Bai　陰白　SP-1
Yin Bao　陰包　LV-9
Yin Du　陰都　KI-19
Yin Gu　陰谷　KI-10
Yin Jiao　陰交　CO-7
Yin Jiao　齦交　GV-28
Yin Lian　陰廉　LV-11
Yin Ling Quan　陰陵泉　SP-9
Yin Men　陰門　BL-51 [37]
Yin Shi　陰市　ST-33
Yin Tang　印堂　M-HN-3
Yin Xi　陰郄　HT-6
Ying Chuang　膺窗　ST-16
Ying Xiang　迎香　LI-20
Yong Quan　涌泉　KI-1
You Men　幽門　KI-21
Yu Ji　魚際　LU-10
Yu Tang　玉堂　CO-18
Yu Yao　魚腰　M-HN-6
Yu Zhen　玉枕　BL-9
Yu Zhong　彧中　KI-26
Yuan Ye　淵腋　GB-22
Yun Men　雲門　LU-2

Z

Zan Zhu　攢竹　BL-2
Ze Qian　澤前　M-UE-32
Ze Xia　澤下　M-UE-31
Zhang Men　章門　LV-13
Zhao Hai　照海　KI-6
Zhe Jin　輒筋　GB-23
Zheng Ying　正營　GB-17
Zhi Bian　秩邊　BL-49 [54]
Zhi Gou　支溝　TW-6
Zhi Shi　志室　BL-47 [52]
Zhi Yang　至陽　GV-9
Zhi Yin　至陰　BL-67
Zhi Zheng　支正　SI-7
Zhong Chong　中衝　PC-9
Zhong Dú　中瀆　GB-32
Zhong Dū　中都　LV-6
Zhong Feng　中封　LV-4
Zhong Fu　中府　LU-1
Zhong Guǎn*　中管　CO-12
Zhong Ji　中極　CO-3
Zhong Liao　中髎　BL-33
Zhong Lu Shu　中膂俞　BL-29
Zhong Shu　中樞　GV-7
Zhong Ting　中庭　CO-16
Zhong Wan　中脘　CO-12
Zhong Zhù　中注　KI-15
Zhong Zhǔ　中渚　TW-3
Zhou Liao　肘髎　LI-12
Zhou Rong　周榮　SP-20
Zhu Bin　築賓　KI-9
Zi Gong　紫宮　CO-19
Zi Gong　子宮　M-CA-18
Zu Lin Qi　足臨泣　GB-41
Zu Qiao Yin　足竅陰　GB-44
Zu San Li　足三里　ST-36
Zu Wu Li　足五里　LV-10
Zuo Gu　坐骨　N-BW-17

FURTHER READING

Philosophy and Religion

Chan, Wing-Tsit, trans. and comp.
A Source Book in Chinese Philosophy.
Princeton NJ: Princeton University Press, 1963.

Earhart, Byron H, edit.
Religious Traditions of the World.
San Francisco: HarperCollins Publishers, 1993.

Smith, Huston.
The Illustrated World's Religions:
A Guide to Our Wisdom Traditions
San Francisco: HarperCollins Publishers, 1994.

Suzuki, D.T,
The Essentials of Zen Buddhism
New York: Greenwood Publishers, 1973 (1962)

Watts, Alan W.
The Way of Zen.
New York: Random House, 1957.

Wong, Eva.
The Shambhala Guide to Taoism.
Boston: Shambhala Publications, 1997.

Zimmer, Heinrich.
Philosophies of India.
Edited by Joseph Campbell.
Princeton NJ: Princeton University Press, 1969.

Western Medicine

Dirix, A., H.G. Knuttgen, and K. Tittel, editors.
Olympic Book of Sports Medicine.
Malden MA: Blackwell Science, 1991 (1988).

Dox, Ida, John Melloni, and Gilbert Eisner.
The HarperCollins Illustrated Medical Dictionary.
New York: HarperCollins Publishers, 1993.

Garrick, James G., and David R. Webb
Sports Injuries: Diagnosis and Management.
Philadelphia: W.B. Saunders Co., 1999 (1990).

Hippocrates.
Hippocrates.
Translated by W.H.S. Jones.
Cambridge MA: Harvard University Press, 1923.

McMinn, R.M.H.
Color Atlas of Human Anatomy. 3rd edition.
London: Mosby Year Book, 1993

Netter, Frank H.
Atlas of Human Anatomy.
Summit, NJ: Novartis Pharmaceuticals, 1989.

Tortora, Gerald.
Principles of Human Anatomy. 8th edition.
New York: HarperCollins Publishers, 1999.

Integrated and Alternative Medicine

Alternative Medicine: Expanding Medical Horizons.
(A Report to the National Institutes of Health on
Alternative Medical Systems and Practices in
the United States.) NIH Publ. No. 94-066.
Washington DC: U.S. Government Printing
Office, 1994.

Maslow, Abraham H.
The Farther Reaches of Human Nature.
New York: Viking Press, 1971.

Moyers, Bill.
Healing and the Mind.
New York: Doubleday, 1993.

Porter, Roy, edit.
Medicine: A History of Healing.
New York: Marlowe & Company, 1997.

Reich, Wilhelm.
Selected Writings: An Introduction to Orgonomy.
New York: Farrar, Straus and Giroux, 1960.

Vogel, Virgil J.
American Indian Medicine.
Normon OK: Univ. of Oklahoma Press, 1970.

Weil, Andrew.
Natural Health, Natural Medicine:
A Comprehensive Manual for
Wellness and Self-Care.
Boston: Houghton Mifflin, 1990.
———. *Health and Healing: Understanding*
Conventional and Alternative Medicine.
Boston: Houghton Mifflin, 1983.

Eastern Medicine

Beinfield, Harriet, and Efrem Korngold.
Between Heaven and Earth:
A Guide to Chinese Medicine.
New York: Ballantine, 1991.

Ellis, Andrew, Nigel Wiseman, and Ken Boss.
Fundamentals of Chinese Acupuncture.
Revised edition. (translation and compilation
from modern and classic Chinese texts).
Brookline MA: Paradigm Publications, 1991.

Ellis, Andrew, and Nigel Wiseman.
The Fundamentals of Chinese Medicine.
Brookline MA: Paradigm Publications, 1985.

Kaptchuk, Ted J.
The Web That Has No Weaver:
Understanding Chinese Medicine.
New York: Congdon & Weed, 1983.

Maciocia, Giovanni.
The Foundations of Chinese Medicine.
London: Churchhill Livingston, 1989.

Shanghai College of Traditional Medicine.
Acupuncture: A Comprehensive Text.
Translated and edited by John O'Connor and Dan
Bensky. Seattle WA: Eastland Press, 1981.

Soulié de Morant, George.
Chinese Acupuncture.
Translated from French by Lawrence Grinnel.
Brookline MA: Paradigm Publications,
English edition 1994, originally published 1950s.

Van Alphen, Jan, and Anthony Aris, editors.
Oriental Medicine: An Illustrated Guide
to the Asian Arts of Healing.
Boston: Shambala Publications, 1997.

Veith, Ilza, trans.
The Yellow Emperor's Classic
of Internal Medicine.
Berkeley and Los Angeles: University of
California Press, 1972 (1949).

Zimmer, Henry R.
Hindu Medicine.
Baltimore: John Hopkins University Press, 1948.

Herbal Medicine

Bensky, Dan, and R. Barolet.
Chinese Herbal Medicine:
Materia Medica.
Seattle WA: Eastland Press, 1993.

Duke, James, and S. Foster.
Peterson's Field Guide to Medicinal Plants.
Boston: Houghton Mifflin, 1990

Grieve, Maude.
A Modern Herbal.
New York: Dover, 1971 (1931)

Healing Arts

Byers, Dwight C.
Better Health with Foot Reflexology:
The Original Inghan Method.
Saint Petersburg, FL: Ingham Publishing, 1983.

Cohen, Kenneth S.
The Way of Qigong: The Art and Science
of Chinese Energy Healing.
New York: Ballantine Books, 1997.

Gach, Michael Reed.
Acupressure's Potent Points:
A Guide to Self-Care.
New York: Bantam, 1990.

Rolf, Ida.
Rolfing: The Integration of Human Structures.
New York: Harper & Row, 1978.

Stillerman, Elaine.
Encyclopedia of Bodywork.
New York: Facts on File, 1996.

Serizawa, Katsusuke.
Tsubo: Vital Points for Oriental Therapy.
Tokyo: Japan Publications, 1976

Teeguarden, Iona Marsaa.
A Complete Guide to Acupressure.
Tokyo: Japan Publications, 1992.

Yang, Jwing-Ming
The Root of Chinese Qigong.
Jamaica Plain, MA: YMAA Publications, 1989.
———. *Chinese Qigong Massage.*
Boston MA: YMAA Publication Center, 1992.

Martial Arts

Draeger, Donn F., and Robert W. Smith
Comprehensive Asian Fighting Arts.
New York: Kodansha, 1980.

Draeger, Donn F.
Classical Budo.
New York: Weatherhill, 1996.

Farkas, Emil, and John Corcoran.
Martial Arts: Traditions, History, People.
New York: Smith Publications, 1983.

Funakoshi, Gichin.
Karate-Do: My Way of Life.
Tokyo: Kodansha, 1975.

Haines, Bruce A.
Karate's History and Traditions.
Tokyo: Tuttle, 1968.

Kano, Jigoro.
Kodokan Judo.
Tokyo: Kodansha, 1986 (1956).

Lee, Bruce.
Tao of Jeet Kune Do.
Santa Clarita, CA: Ohara Publications, 1975.

Nelson, Randy F., edit.
The Overlook Martial Arts Reader:
Classic Writings on Philosophy and Technique.
Woodstock NY: Overlook Press, 1989.

Tedeschi, Marc.
Hapkido: Traditions, Philosophy, Technique.
New York: Weatherhill, Fall 2000.

Tohei, Koichi.
Aikido: The Arts of Self Defense.
New York: Japan Publications, 1963.

Ueshiba, Morihei.
Budo: Teachings of the Founder of Aikido.
Tokyo: Kodansha, 1991 (1938).